SALMONELLOSIS

MICROBIOLOGIC, PATHOLOGIC AND CLINICAL FEATURES

Robert H. Rubin, M.D.

Assistant Professor of Medicine, Harvard Medical School; Assistant Physician, Infectious Disease Unit, Massachusetts General Hospital, Boston, Mass.

Louis Weinstein, M.D.

Physician, Peter Bent Brigham Hospital; Visiting Professor of Medicine, Harvard Medical School, Boston, Mass.

Stratton Intercontinental Medical Book Corporation
New York

Stratton Intercontinental Medical Book Corp.
381 Park Avenue South / New York, N.Y. 10016

LC 77-23960 / ISBN 0-913258-51-2

Printed in U.S.A

Contents

Foreword

Salmonellae are among the most resourceful and successful of human pathogens, and as such have long beguiled microbiologists, epidemiologists, and clinicians. Bacteria of this genus, extensively distributed in animal reservoirs, have shown a phenomenal capacity to adapt, for self-perpetuation, to newer mass production technics of our society, whether in the processing of food, the preparaion of pharmaceuticals, or commercial raising of pet turtles. In view of the ubiquity of these organisms, the fact that salmonella infections are quite common is not as surprising, perhaps, as the fact that such infections are not universal. Further enhancing the challenge these organisms offer to medicine and public health is their versatility and capacity to undergo genetic change by varied mechanisms. Based on analyses of somatic (O) and flagellar (H) antigens, there are approximately 1300 different serotypes in this genus, and there is no reason to believe the limit has been reached. Lysogenic conversion, in which infection by a specific phage causes change in an O antigen characteristic of one salmonella serotype to that characteristic of another serotype, adds complexity to an already difficult identification problem. But this is not all! These bacteriologic masters of disguise have, on very rare occasions, even attempted to cloak themselves in anonymity through the acquisition of a lac^+ plasmid (conferring the capacity to ferment lactose), and become lost in the crowd among the fecal flora under scrutiny in the Diagnostic Microbiology Laboratory. In recent years more threatening plasmids (R-plasmids mediating resistance to chloramphenicol and ampicillin) have appeared increasingly among the *Enterobacteriaceae,* including the *Salmonellae*.

A lucid overview of the fascinating microbiologic and epidemiologic attributes of these organisms is presented in the first two chapters of this monograph by Drs. Rubin and Weinstein. Information of particular relevance to the internist and infectious disease specialist is featured; and, appropriately, emphasis is placed on the epidemiologic value of serotyping in the recognition of less obvious outbreaks and in the identification of their sources. For example, reference is made to the international outbreak a decade ago of sporadic cases of salmonellosis due to an unusual serotype (*S. cubana*). Because of the uniqueness of this antigenic type it could be identified among a background of infections due to more common serotypes. In this way contamination of the crude red dye ("cochineal") with salmonella was eventually pinpointed, and the route of clinical infection via commercial carmine red dyes was uncovered.

The wide spectrum of disease syndromes produced by salmonellae can be considered as the clinical counterpart of their microbiologic diversity. The major portion of this monograph is devoted to the clinical features of salmonellosis. The pathogenesis of the common (gastroenteritis, intestinal carrier state) and the less common (enteric fever) forms of infection with this organism is well described. Helpful guidelines are offered for treatment (and just as important, for "non-treatment") of salmonella gastroenteritis and the intestinal carrier state. Typhoid fever, one of the common infectious diseases in this country early in this century, is now a rarity. It is still common in other parts of the world, however, and American travelers and new immigrants continue to serve as sources for introduction of fresh cases. The recent extension of typhoid fever (due to chloramphenicol-resistant *S. typhi*) from Mexico, where a major epidemic occurred, to California is a clear example cited by the authors. The detailed description of this disease as it now presents, and a consideration of the problem of the chronic typhoid carrier state, are important elements in this review. The extensive experience of the authors in infectious disease provides a solid basis for their descriptions and review of the many unusual salmonella syndromes (bacteremia, endocarditis, endaortitis, vertebral osteomyelitis, etc.) which may not be so familiar to many physicians. The "mini" case reports included in their review demonstrate in concrete terms many of the problems in diagnosis and treatment of salmonellosis. Dr. Louis Weinstein has had a long and continuing interest in salmonella infections. (I can still recall, many years ago as a resident, his insistence on our searching for an aortic aneurysm in an elderly patient with cryptogenic persistent *Salmonella cholerasuis* bacteremia; and, indeed, such an infected aneurysm was found and proved to be the focus for the bacteremia.)

No consideration of salmonellae would be complete without recording their traits as "opportunists" in patients with hemoglobinopathies and other hemolytic anemias, and in patients with schistosomiasis, neoplastic disease, etc.; and these aspects are fully discussed by the authors in the clinical section of this monograph. Of interest to the practicing physician will be the detailed appraisal of the various current antimicrobial drugs in the treatment of salmonellosis, particularly in view of the increasing emergence of R-plasmids.

This monograph, directed toward the internist and the infectious disease specialist, provides a thorough, well-referenced, authoritative evaluation of the "current status of the field," with regard to salmonella infections.

Morton N. Swartz, M.D.

CHAPTER I

Microbiologic Characteristics of the Salmonella

Bacteria of the genus *Salmonella* are perhaps the most ubiquitous pathogens in nature, affecting, in a worldwide distribution, not only man and his domestic animals, but also reptiles, wild mammals, birds, and even insects. Salmonellae are closely related biochemically to *Arizona* and *Citrobacter*. These genera form one of the six major divisions (tribes) of the family *Enterobacteriaceae*. The salmonellae are classified in three primary species: *Salmonella choleraesuis, Salmonella typhi,* and *Salmonella enteritidis*. *S. choleraesuis* and *S. typhi* each consist of a single serotype (subtype). In contrast, over 1400 antigenically distinct serotypes of *S. enteritidis* have been defined. Many of them are highly adapted to specific ecologic niches, and tend to produce specific clinical syndromes. The "formal" taxonomic designation of these serotypes is illustrated by the following: *S. enteritidis* serotype newport, *S. enteritidis* serotype paratyphi, *S. enteritidis* serotype enteritidis, etc. [1,2]. However, by convention and for convenience, this somewhat awkward formality is usually bypassed in favor of the traditional system of using just the name of the genus and serotype to designate these organisms, as in the following: *S. newport, S. paratyphi, S. enteritidis,* etc. This simpler nomenclature is employed in this monograph.

Ecologic Divisions

More useful to the clinician than the species divisions of the salmonellae is a consideration of the ecologic divisions into which they may be placed on the basis of host preferences and adaptations [2]:

(A) *Salmonella serotypes highly adapted to man include S. typhi, S. paratyphi,* S. schottmülleri,* S. hirschfeldi* and S. sendai.* There is no zoonotic reservoir for these organisms; animal infection is rare and accidental,

* These three salmonella serotypes were formerly designated *S. paratyphi A, S. paratyphi B,* and *S. paratyphi C,* respectively.

and human-to-human transmission is critical in the epidemiology of the diseases they produce.

(B) *Salmonella serotypes highly adapted to specific non-human hosts.* Each domestic farm animal has its own host-adapted serotype (fowl, *S. pullorum* and *S. gallinarum*; cattle, *S. dublin*; horses, *S. abortusequi*; sheep, *S. abortusovis*; swine, *S. choleraesuis* and *S. typhisuis*). With the exception of *S. dublin* and *S. choleraesuis,* the other species uncommonly produce human disease in man, require a large inoculum to produce infection, and rarely are responsible for more than a self-limited gastroenteritis in man.

(C) *Salmonella serotypes unadapted to specific hosts.* The other 1400 serotypes ubiquitous in nature belong in this category. They share the following characteristics: They usually produce acute gastroenteritis (food-poisoning) of short duration (a few days) after a short incubation period (12–48 hrs.); they invade the bloodstream uncommonly; relatively large numbers of organisms are necessary to produce disease. These species are involved in >80% of the salmonella infections that presently occur in the United States.

Bacteriologic Considerations

Salmonellae are gram-negative, flagellated, nonencapsulated, nonsporulating, aerobic (facultatively anaerobic*) bacilli (Fig. 1). Like other *Enterobacteriaceae,* they form relatively large, shiny, grey colonies on standard blood agar media, and are distinguished from one another by a complex scheme of biochemical tests. A simplified version is illustrated in Table 1. The technics employed in the culture and isolation of strains that are to be speciated are complex and variable and depend, in large part, upon the sites being cultured for these organisms and the availability of the diagnostic laboratory. A few simple rules are helpful to keep in mind.

When culture of a normally sterile site such as blood, cerebrospinal fluid, joint, etc., is carried out, selective media are *not* required. Nonselective or enriched ones (blood or chocolate agar or nutrient broth) that support the growth of any of the common aerobic bacterial pathogens are adequate for primary isolation of these organisms.

When salmonella invade the gastrointestinal tract, culture of from 5 to 10 gram aliquots of feces is far more efficient than rectal swabs in detecting the presence of the causative bacteria. Multiple specimens (at least three individual stools) should be cultured in these cases, because this appreciably increases the possibility of establishing the diagnosis. Feces obtained during the active or acute phase of the disease are more likely to yield salmonellae because they are present in much larger numbers during the period of active disease than during the convalescent phase of illness.

* Recently, there has been a report by Huber et al. [3] of an unusual *S. typhi* that grew only under anerobic conditions when first isolated from blood culture, and required several passages before reversion to the usual facultative state; this behavior is most atypical of salmonellae.

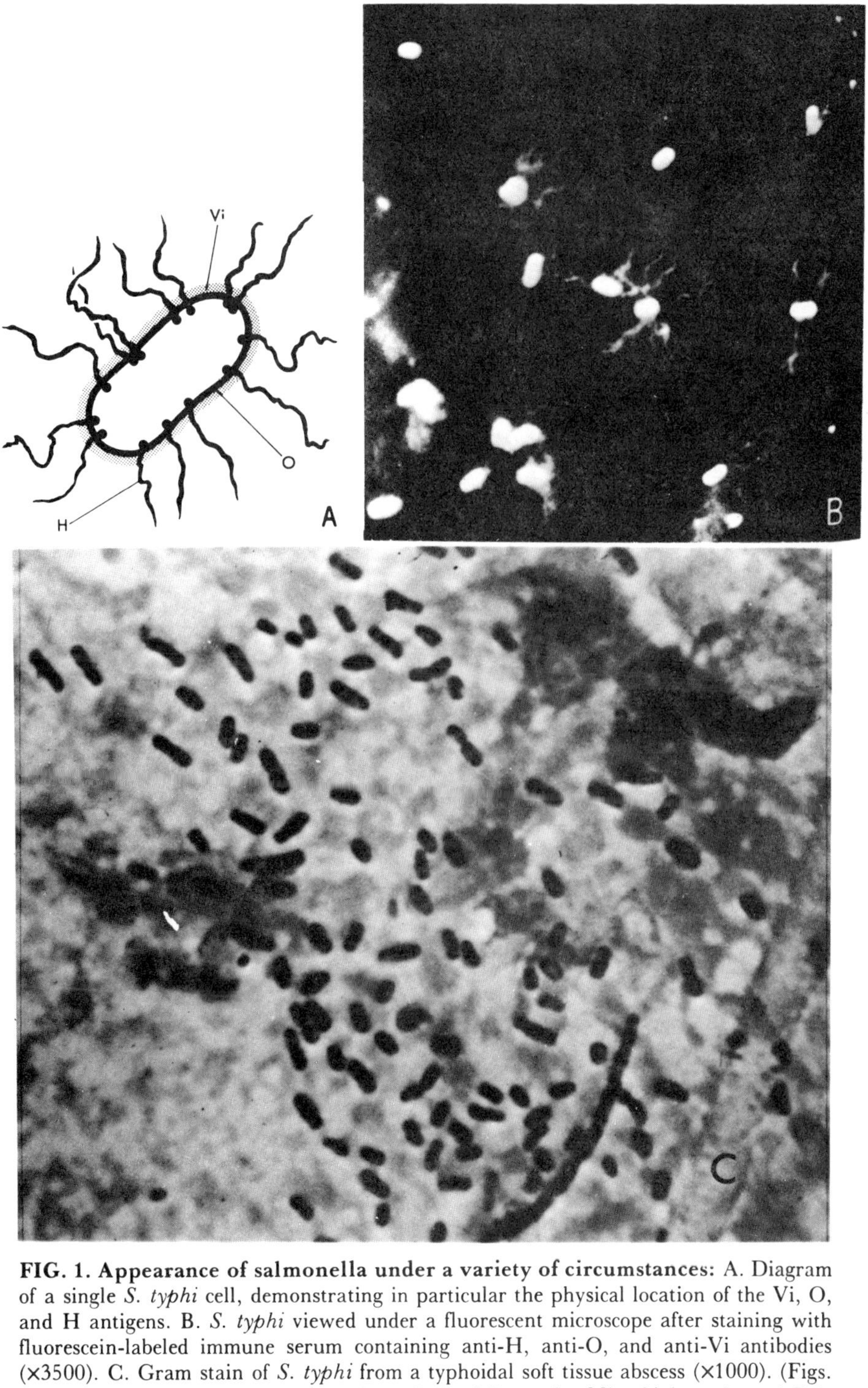

FIG. 1. Appearance of salmonella under a variety of circumstances: A. Diagram of a single *S. typhi* cell, demonstrating in particular the physical location of the Vi, O, and H antigens. B. *S. typhi* viewed under a fluorescent microscope after staining with fluorescein-labeled immune serum containing anti-H, anti-O, and anti-Vi antibodies (×3500). C. Gram stain of *S. typhi* from a typhoidal soft tissue abscess (×1000). (Figs. 1A and B are from Sonnenwirth AC, in Davis BD, et al.: *Microbiology,* Second Edition, Harper and Row, New York, 1973, p. 760 [8].)

TABLE 1. Differentiation of Some of the Enterobacteriaceae by Biochemical Tests (modified from Ewing, WH: Enteric Bacteriology Laboratoriess, DHEW-PHS-CDC, Atlanta, Georgia, 30333, July, 1973)

	Salmonella species	Escherichia coli	Shigella species	Klebsiella pneumoniae	Enterobacter cloacae	Serratia marcescens	Proteus mirabilis
Indol	−	+	− or +	−	−	−	−
Methyl red	+	+	+	− or +	−	− or +	+
Voges-Proskauer	−	−	−	+	+	+	− or +
Simmons' citrate	d	−	−	+	+	+	+ or (+)
Hydrogen sulfide (TSI)	+	−	−	−	−	−	+
Urease	−	−	−	+	+ or −	d^w	+
KCN	−	−	−	+	+	+	+
Motility	+	+ or −	−	−	+	+	+
Gelatin (22 C)	−	−	−	−	(+) or −	+ or (+)	+
Lysine decarboxylase	+	d	−	+	−	+	−
Arginine dihydrolase	+ or (+)	d	d	−	+	−	−
Ornithine decarboxylase	+	d	d	−	+	+	+
Phenylalanine deaminase	−	−	−	−	−	−	+
Malonate	−	−	−	+	+ or −	−	−
Gas from glucose	+	+	−	+	+	+ or −	+
Lactose	−	+	−	+	+ or (+)	−	−
Sucrose	−	d	−	+	+	+	d
Mannitol	+	+	+ or −	+	+	+	−
Dulcitol	d	d	d	− or +	− or +	−	−
Salicin	−	d	−	+	+ or (+)	+	d
Adonitol	−	−	−	+ or −	− or +	d	−
Inositol	d	−	−	+	d	d	−
Sorbitol	+	d	d	+	+	+	−
Arabinose	+	+	d	+	+	−	−
Raffinose	−	d	d	+	+	−	−
Rhamnose	+	d	d	+	+	−	−

Key: + = 90% or more positive in 1 or 2 days
− = 90% or more negative
d = may be positive or negative
w = weakly positive
(+) = delayed positive
+ or − = majority of cultures positive

A variety of media are available for *transport* of stool specimens. In addition, *enrichment* media may be used to increase the yield of organisms over that obtained by direct plating of feces, and *selective* ones to suppress the multiplication of members of the "normal" intestinal microflora and to permit differentiation of those that grow from salmonella. The current recommendations of the Center for Disease Control for isolation of salmonellae are presented in Table 2. *Transport* media are of greatest value in field surveys, epidemiologic investigations, or other circumstances in which stools are obtained at a distance from a diagnostic laboratory, but they are not usually used within a hospital setting. Many laboratories often culture feces directly on *selective* media the day that a specimen is received; a tube of *enrichment* medium is heavily inoculated at the same time, incubated overnight, and then plated. These technics increase the likelihood of distinguishing salmonellae from the very large number of organisms that make up the normal microbial population of the intestinal tract [4,5].

Salmonella Antigens and Their Importance

Of great clinical interest and importance are the methods employed for speciation of the salmonellae. The "O" (somatic) and "H" (flagellar) antigens of specific salmonella can be identified by the use of highly purified antisera (Fig. 1). Nine serogroups (A to I) of this genus have been identified, using the Kauffman-White scheme, on the basis of their somatic antigens. Although a single species may contain several O antigens, each always has a specific component For example, Group A always contains type 2, group B type 4, Group C type 6, group D type 9, etc. Specific species within each O group are defined in terms of the H antigens. One of two kinds of these H antigens, phase 1 or 2, may be present in a given strain at different times. Phase 1 is shared by only a few species of salmonella, while phase 2 is more widely distributed and less specific. The formation of phase antigen is genetically controlled; one or both phases may be detected in cultured cells. Although *S. typhi* and *S. enteritidis* both belong to group D and contain O antigens 9 and 12, the flagellar (H) antigen of the former is *d,* and that of the latter is *g,m* [6–8]. Rare, newly-discovered serotypes may not fit into this scheme. However, these are involved in human infections uncommonly, as serogroups A–E are responsible for >90% of the disease in man. The antigenic composition of some of the more common serotypes of the genus *Salmonella* are listed in Table 3.

In addition to their clinical and microbiologic importance, the H and O antigens are very helpful markers in studies of the epidemiology of salmonellosis in large populations as well as in single individuals. Specific serotypes are associated with particular modes of spread of the organisms and with the type of disease that develops. Other technics of value for large-scale epidemiologic investigations include fluorescent antibody staining for rapid

TABLE 2. Recommended Transport, Enrichment, and Plating Media to be Employed in the Isolation of Salmonellae from Fecal Specimens*

Etiology	Transport Media	Enrichment Media	Plating Media	Remarks
S. typhi	1. Buffered Glycerol saline 2. Amies 3. Stuart's 4. Cary-Blair	1. Selenite 2. Tetrathionate	1. Bismuth Sulfite Agar 2. Salmonella-Shigella Agar 3. MacConkey Agar	Direct plating of fresh stool specimen preferred
Non-typhoidal salmonellae	1. Tetrathionate Brilliant Green Broth 2. Buffered Glycerol Saline 3. Cary-Blair 4. Amies' 5. Stuart's	1. Tetrathionate Brilliant Green Broth 2. Selenite Broth 3. Tetrathionate Broth	1. Brilliant Green Agar 2. Bismuth Sulfite Agar 3. Salmonella-Shigella Agar 4. Xylose-Lysine-Deoxy-cholate Agar	May be transported in enrichment broth.

* As prepared by Morris, GK and Mackel, DC, Epidemiological Services Laboratory, Bacterial Diseases Branch, Bureau of Epidemiology, Center for Disease Control, Atlanta, Georgia. The media are listed in order of preference. For details on the constitution of these media, the reader is referred to Buchanan RE, Gibbons NE: *Bergey's Manual of Determinative Bacteriology* (8th ed.), Baltimore: Williams and Wilkins, 1974.

TABLE 3. Kauffmann-White Classification of Common Salmonella Serotypes (modified from Bowmer [6])

Serotype	Group	O Antigens	H. Antigens	
			Phase 1	Phase 2
S. paratyphi A	A	(1)*, _2_**, 12	a	—
S. schottmülleri	B	1, _4_, (5), 12	b	1, 2
S. typhimurium	B	1, _4_, (5), 12	(i)	1, 2
S. heidelberg	B	1, _4_, 5, 12	r	1, 2
S. canada	B	_4_, 12	b	1, 6
S. saint-paul	B	1, _4_, 5, 12	e, h	1, 2
S. hirschfeldi	C_1	_6_, 7	c	1, 5
S. bareilly	C_1	_6_, 7	y	1, 5
S. choleraesuis	C_1	_6_, 7	c	1, 5
S. montevideo	C_1	_6_, 7	g, m, s	—
S. oranienburg	C_1	_6_, 7	m, t	—
S. newport	C_2	_6_, 8	(e, h)	1, 2
S. typhi	D	_9_, 12	d	—
S. enteritidis	D	1, _9_, 12	g, m	—
S. pullorum/gallinarum	D	(1), _9_, 12	—	—
S. anatum	E	_3_, 10	e, h	1, 6
S. vancouver	I	_16_	c	1, 5

* Parentheses indicate that antigenic determinant may be absent or difficult to detect.
** Italicized number signifies major determinant of group.

identification of salmonellae in fecal specimens, and phage-typing. The latter is currently available for only a few species, chiefly *S. typhi*, *S. schottmulleri* and *S. typhimurium*. These methods are of limited usefulness in the care and evaluation of individual cases of infection.

Measurement of agglutinating antibodies against the *O* and *H* antigens of the typhoid bacillus was introduced by Widal in 1896 [9]. Attempts have been made to expand the usefulness of this procedure by the use of additional antigens (the O antigens of salmonella Groups A–E, and the H antigens of the paratyphoid species). However, salmonella gastroenteritis and the carrier state do not induce much antibody response; this limits the clinical application of the test primarily to the enteric fevers [10,11], and, perhaps, to long-standing smouldering infections such as osteomyelitis. Traditionally, a serologic diagnosis of typhoid fever is made on the basis of either a four-fold rise in the titer of antibody to the O antigen or a titer of >1 : 50 or 1 : 100 in a single specimen studied in the first two or three weeks of illness in an unimmunized individual [12]. However, in some cases of untreated typhoid fever an increase in the level of this antibody does not occur [13], and treatment with effective antimicrobial agents may blunt the immunologic response. Titration of the level of antibody for H antigen is of little value in the diagnosis of active salmonella infection since an increase may be detected in other types of inflammatory response [12]. Administration of typhoid vaccine leads to an increase in both anti-O and anti-H antibodies; the former falls after several months; the latter may persist, at lower but possibly significant levels for years [12,14,15].

It has recently become apparent that infections with other Group D salmonellae, such as *S. javiana* and *S. enteritidis,* and even with species that do not belong in this group, such as *S. typhimurium* (Group B), can occasionally produce "diagnostic" changes in the level of agglutinating antibody for the typhoid O antigen [16,17]. Similar false positive increases have been reported in patients with chronic active liver disease and other inflammatory disorders featured by elevations of immunoglobulin [18]. It is apparent that the time-honored agglutination tests for the diagnosis of disease due to salmonella constitute a rather poor approach to the diagnosis of disease caused by this group of organisms. Only increasing or high levels of antibody to somatic antigens are of any value. The primary specific diagnostic method is isolation and identification of the organism.

The O or lipopolysaccharide (LPS) somatic antigen appears to be an important determinant of the virulence of salmonellae. "Rough" mutants of organisms that lack the O-specific sidechains of the LPS are nonpathogenic; "semi-rough" strains in which the length of the polymer is shortened are only moderately invasive; "smooth" ones, characterized by the presence of an intact sidechain, are highly pathogenic [19,20]. A recent study of strains of *S. typhimurium* differing only in their content of O-antigen by Makela et al. [21] indicated the following: strains containing antigens 4 and 12 were highly virulent; those with O-antigens 9 and 12 were less pathogenic and those with O-antigens 6 and 7 were essentially noninvasive. These observations suggested that differences in the structure of O-antigen (substitution of one sugar molecule for another—abequose for 4,12 vs. tyvelose for 9,12) play an important part in determining the recognition of the organism by either the immune system or functioning phagocytes, or both. Strains that are readily controlled by host defense mechanisms are of low pathogenicity; those in which the antigenic composition effectively protects the invading salmonellae from recognition by the host are highly successful pathogens.

A third antigen, the polysaccharide *Vi,* may form an outer coat that covers the somatic antigens (Fig. 1). *Vi* is commonly present in *S. hirschfeldi* (*paratyphi C*) and *S. typhi.* This antigen appears to interfere with the activity of bactericidal antibody and phagocytosis both *in vitro* and *in vivo.* The presence or absence of Vi in these two species has been correlated with virulence [22–24]. Anti-Vi agglutinins appear late in the course of typhoid fever, usually disappear with recovery and are unaltered by immunization [12,25,26]. The anti-Vi reaction has been proposed as a screening test for typhoid carriers. However, an incidence of false positive and false negative reactions of 6–8% and 30%, respectively, has limited its applicability [12,25,26].

The O antigens, unlike the H and Vi, are part of a macromolecular structure that forms the outer portion of the cell wall of salmonella and possesses important biologic properties. This complex is *endotoxin* or lipopolysaccharide (LPS) and is made up of three layers; an outer (O-polysaccharide), middle (R-core) and basal (Lipid A) (Fig. 2). The *O-polysaccharide* is composed of a regular sequence of repeating sugars on the surface of the cell wall that determines the specific nature of the O antigen. The *R-core* serves to link the O-polysaccharide to the lipid moiety, and contains five sugars, phosphate and

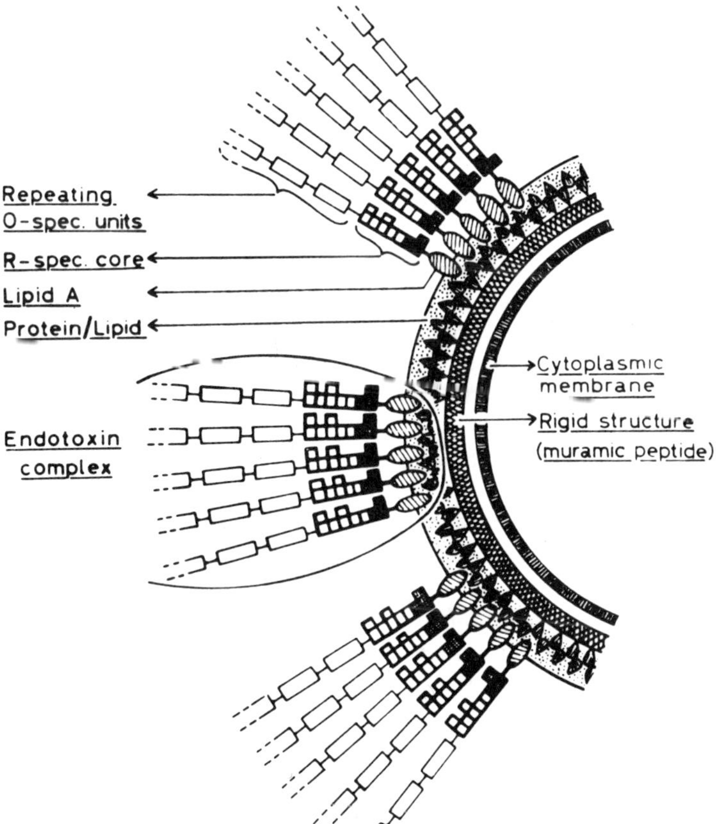

FIG. 2. Schematic diagram of the cell wall of the salmonellae and other Enterobacteriaceae. (From Wilson GS, Miles A: *Topley and Wilson's Principles of Bacteriology, Virology and Immunity,* Sixth Edition, Williams and Wilkins, Baltimore, 1975, p. 363.)

O-phosphorylethanolamine. Recent studies [27] have indicated that antibodies directed against elements of the R-core protect against infections caused by a wide variety of gram-negative bacteria. *Lipid A* binds the entire endotoxin molecule to the rest of the cell wall structure; it is a complex of repeating fatty acid-containing diglucosamine units attached to amino and hydroxyl units [8,28,29].

The biologic effects of endotoxin are of great importance to the clinician because one or more of them may play a role in the morbidity and mortality associated with infection due to enterobacteria, in general, and salmonella, in particular. The clinical effects of this compound are discussed in detail in Chapters III and IV. The complex LPS macromolecule produces fever, interacts with the formed elements of the blood, triggers the complement and clotting cascades, alters host resistance, resets hormonal and metabolic millieu, and is responsible for many of the clinical features of "septic shock." The role played by endotoxin in infections caused by intact microorganisms [8,28,29] is discussed below.

Plasmids and Salmonellae

Over the past three decades there has been an explosion of interest in *plasmids,* small, self-replicating extrachromosomal elements that carry genetic information from one bacterium to another.* To the clinician concerned with the management of serious enterobacterial infections, including those caused by salmonella, the plasmids of greatest interest are those that mediate antibiotic resistance—the *resistance plasmids* (*R plasmids*) or *R-factors.* These are composed of two elements: (a) the *resistance transfer factor* (RTF) which initiates bacterial conjugation and the exchange of genetic material, and (b) the *resistance determinant,* which contains the genes coding for resistance to an antimicrobial drug. Other genetic information may be carried by the R-factor; this includes resistance to bacterial killing by a variety of metal ions [30,31]. The potential importance of these two types of genetic information is demonstrated by a recent report [32] of an outbreak of *Salmonella typhimurium* infection among burned patients. This organism carried R plasmid-mediated resistance not only to ampicillin, chloramphenicol, tetracycline, streptomycin and sulfonamides, but also to silver nitrate and mercuric chloride. The lack of sensitivity to silver nitrate was of particular importance because of the use of this compound to prevent bacterial colonization and invasion of the burned surfaces. This experience, and many others involving infections caused

* Plasmids that replicate either separately from the host chromosome or integrated into it are known as episomes. Although the terms plasmid and episome have been used interchangeably in the past, the term episome is now restricted only to those plasmids with the two properties described above [30,31].

by plasmid-mediated antibiotic resistance in salmonella, underscores the fact that once a new R-factor is formed or introduced into a susceptible bacterial population, there is an initial high frequency of transfer of the plasmid, particularly when there is selection pressure for resistance to a particular antibiotic because of exposure to the agent (see Chapter II).

Plasmid incompatibility is defined as a situation in which two different plasmids are unable to coexist in the same host cell in the absence of selection pressures. Groups of plasmids that are mutually incompatible can be defined. This phenomenon is useful in the study of the characteristics and mechanisms of R-plasmid-mediated resistance to antibiotics [31].

That R-factor-mediated resistance to antimicrobial agents is of great clinical importance is emphasized by a large number of observations.

Epidemics of typhoid fever due to chloramphenicol-resistant *S. typhi* have occurred in several areas of the world, including Latin America, India, and Southeast Asia [33–36]. Resistance to this drug, when examined in strains responsible for these outbreaks, has been shown to be transmitted by plasmids; all of the R-factors identified belong to plasmid incompatibility Group H [36]. Of great concern has been the report of the isolation of a strain of *S. typhi* not susceptible to either ampicillin or chloramphenicol. This was isolated from an individual with typhoid fever acquired in Mexico. The patient was treated with ampicillin, but during the course of therapy the organism developed resistance to this agent, as a result of acquisition of an additional R-factor that was in incompatibility Group I and coded for resistance to both ampicillin and kanamycin. It was distinct from and quite compatible with the Group H plasmid already present that determined lack of susceptibility to chloramphenicol [36,37]. Similar strains of the organism with the same genetic markers have been recovered from cases of typhoid fever in Mexico [38]. The epidemiologic significance of these findings is discussed in Chapter II.

R-plasmid-transmitted antibiotic resistance has also been demonstrated in species of salmonella responsible for nontyphoidal salmonella infection in the United States and Europe [39–52]. Until recently, *S. typhimurium* was the serotype that exhibited plasmid-mediated resistance to one or more antimicrobial agents most often. Recent studies [49,50] have indicated that the frequency of strains of this organism resistant to antimicrobial agents has been increasing: 49% of strains isolated in California [49] and 57% of those recovered in the northeastern United States [50] are of this type. However, other rather common serotypes, including *S. heidelberg* (57% resistant in California, 36% in the Northeast), *S. newport* (43% in California, 30% in the Northeast), *S. saint-paul* (40% in California, 16% in the Northeast), and *S. derby* (29% in the Northeast), are manifesting increasing levels of resistance to antibiotics [49,50]. From 70 to 90% of this resistance is mediated by plasmids [39–50]. In contrast, *S. infantis* and *S. enteritidis,* two other common serotypes, remain highly sensitive to antibacterial drugs. There is no adequate explanation for the variation in susceptibility to antibiotics among different serotypes of the salmonella. It has been postulated that there may be a difference in the susceptibility to the entrance or perpetuation of R-factors that determine resistance, possibly because of subtle changes in the composition of bacterial cell wall, incompatibility, restriction of DNA or inhibition of transcription or translocation [31,49,53,54].

CHAPTER II

Epidemiology of Disease Caused by Salmonella

The annual incidence of isolations of salmonellae in the United States is approximately 10–12 per 100,000 population. However, investigation of several large epidemics has suggested that the number of unreported cases is quite large, the true annual incidence probably being about 100 times (two million cases per year) that reported [2,55,56]. The frequency of both *S. typhi* and nontyphoidal salmonella infections reaches a peak in the summer months in the United States, although a substantial number of cases occur throughout the year. The highest incidence occurs in the summer and fall, and correlates with outbreaks of food poisoning during this time, also perhaps with an increase in person-to-person transmission, especially in children [2,57–59]. There is no sex preponderance. Age-specific attack rates for salmonellosis are highest in the age groups under 20 and over 70, and are maximal in infants under one year of age (approximately 130 isolates per 100,000 population) [56]. A case-fatality rate of approximately 0.2% has been observed in epidemics of the disease. The great majority of the deaths occur in infants, among the elderly, and in patients severely ill with other diseases, especially cancer [2]. Once a strain of salmonella has infected one member of a household, there is an approximately 60% chance that at least one other person in the family will develop disease [60]; 20–35% of household contacts of the index case become infected [56,60,61]. About 55% of salmonella isolations are said to be from sporadic cases, 20% from outbreaks in families, 15% from infection of large groups, and 10% from hospitalized patients. However, when intensive epidemiologic investigation has been carried out, it is evident that the majority of cases probably represent unrecognized epidemics in one of the categories described above, rather than isolated cases [2].

There were 5,595 cases of typhoid fever and less than 1,000 cases of other types of salmonellosis recognized in the United States in 1942 [55]. The situation was reversed during the next 3 decades, so that by 1974 only 582 cases of typhoid fever, but 23,838 instances of other types of disease caused by salmonella, were recorded [56]. A similar experience has been noted in other industrialized societies. As the predominant form of disease has changed, so has its epidemiology. While illness produced by *S. typhi* occurs almost exclusively in man, most other serotypes of salmonella are more ubiquitous. A diagnosis of a case of typhoid fever means that the source was a human and that spread to the case was by direct contact or indirectly via contaminated food or water. There must be a human carrier of the organism at some point in the epidemiologic cycle [62]. In contrast, although person-to-person transmission and human carriers of salmonella may play a role in the epidemiology of nontyphoidal salmonella, the most important vehicle is contaminated food [55,56].

EPIDEMIOLOGY OF TYPHOID FEVER

Typhoid fever usually follows the ingestion of drinking water contaminated by feces containing *S. typhi,* or food prepared or handled by a person or persons who are excreting the organisms in their stool and do not wash their hands adequately. Direct transmission from one individual to another may occur via the fecal-oral route, particularly in children because of their relatively poor attention to personal hygiene. It has also been recognized that oysters may be contaminated in polluted river beds, and that flies and dust physically transporting the bacteria may be sources of infection in endemic areas [63]. Large-scale epidemics of typhoid fever in industrial societies have been traced to human fecal contamination of milk products [64,65], spaghetti [66] and corned beef [67–72]. However, poor sanitary practice resulting in wholesale contamination of drinking water by feces containing typhoid bacilli appears to be the major factor involved in major outbreaks of disease due to this organism in the United States [73]. Experiences over the last decade have underscored this point and demonstrated that high mobility and industrialization have increased the opportunity for spread of typhoid disease.

Five-hundred and four cases of typhoid fever discovered in Aberdeen, Scotland in 1964 were associated with ingestion of tinned corned beef shipped to Britain from Argentina [67–72]. Contamination of the meat occurred in Argentina, where river water containing unprocessed sewage was used to cool the containers *after* sterilization. The water seeped through the seams in the cans and reached their contents. Infections in Aberdeen developed not only in individuals who ate the corned beef, but also in those who partook of other meat that became contaminated when cut by the machine that had been used to slice the corned beef [68]. *S. typhi* has never been isolated from raw meat. This reflects the high degree of adaptation of the organism to human hosts, and makes it clear that contamination of meat products takes place only via the secondary contamination that occurs during the manufacturing, packing, or distributing processes [69]. That this course of events is not unusual is emphasized by the fact that at least six other such outbreaks related to corned beef [69–71] had been recognized previously in the United Kingdom.

In the early 1970's, a large-scale epidemic of typhoid fever (>10,000 cases) due to a chloramphenicol-resistant strain occurred in Mexico, an area in which endemic infection is ordinarily common [33,74–77]. As with the disease previously present, contaminated water played the most important role in transmission of the drug-resistant organism [74]. The lack of susceptibility of this strain of *S. typhi* to chloramphenicol was responsible for death among many patients who were treated with this antibiotic before it became apparent that it was ineffective. The specific nature of the drug-resistance provided an excellent epidemiologic marker for infections caused by this strain of *S. typhi*. The Mexican organism was found to be responsible for typhoid fever in Switzerland [75], the United Kingdom [76], the United States [77] and other parts of the world. In Los Angeles, the incidence of this disease, which had been stable for about 15 years, doubled in 1972, and appeared to be showing a tendency to increase beyond this [34]. One-third of the isolates were resistant to chloramphenicol. This outbreak underscores the fact that the mobility of modern society contributes greatly to the spread of typhoid fever to areas far removed from the site of the initially-documented cases and that poor sanitary practice may be the initiating and continuing factor. Recent reports [35,36] of the isolation of chloramphenicol-resistant strains of *S. typhi* in Southeast Asia suggest that this may remain a problem for some time.

The basis for the resistance of the Mexican strain of *S. typhi* to chloramphenicol is a plasmid. The mechanics for selection and transmission from one organism to another of plasmid-mediated resistance to antibiotics have been clearly and succinctly defined by Anderson [36].

> The subject of R-factor-mediated drug resistance in enterobacteria in general, and in pathogenic enterobacteria in particular, can now be viewed in perspective, because much work has been done in this field since R-factors were first discovered. It has been established that these plasmids are now abundant in the enterobacteria of man and livestock throughout the world. This massive shift in the ecology of the enterobacteria of man is the result of the use of antibacterial drugs for the treatment of disease in man caused by enterobacterial and other, often unidentified, pathogens. In animals it is the consequence of the use of antibiotics as feed additives and for the prophylaxis and treatment of disease. Moreover, it is now clear that the R-factors in man and animals are drawn from a common pool.
>
> The enterobacteria in which transferable drug resistance first emerges are ordinary intestinal commensals such as *E. coli*. They are usually nonpathogenic but are highly communicable. They therefore spread to the intestine of other human or animal hosts, irrespective of the use of antibiotics, but their prevalence is sustained by the incessant use of these drugs. From time to time their resistance is transferred to a pathogen which subsequently causes an outbreak of infection. The result is an epidemic of a disease which is no longer susceptible to drugs that might formerly have been used for its treatment. The widespread appearance of chloramphenicol-resistant typhoid fever,

of intractable and virulent outbreaks of infection with multiresistant salmonellae in pediatric units in South America and elsewhere, of epidemic drug-resistant *Shigella dysenteriae* infection in Central America, and of problems of hospital infection with resistant opportunist enterobacterial pathogens in many countries, are worrying examples of this. But such events were predictable, and are yet another warning that rationalization and reduction of the use of antibiotics and other antibacterial drugs are necessary, not only in the developing countries but in the world at large. The medical and veterinary professions bear a heavy responsibility in this respect, as do pharmaceutical manufacturers, who should be watchful for the misuse of their products, and should conduct promotional campaigns with a real awareness of the dangers arising from their abuse. The time has clearly come when international cooperation at legislative and professional levels is needed to attempt to reverse the change in the ecology of the enterobacteria and other organisms that has resulted from the indiscriminate use of antibacterial drugs.

Although the most striking example of this phenomenon is the resistance of *S. typhi* to chloramphenicol, similar observations have been made with respect to resistance to ampicillin among the salmonella that do not cause typhoid fever. Fully 18% of these organisms recently isolated in the northeastern United States have failed to exhibit sensitivity to this form of penicillin. Among the most common serotypes in this group have been *S. typhimurium, S. newport* and *S. heidelberg;* 37, 32, and 30%, respectively, were resistant to the drug [50]. Principles similar to those determining chloramphenicol-resistance of *S. typhi* are involved in the appearance of resistance to ampicillin in other serotypes of salmonella. Selection pressures produced by widespread use of ampicillin in environments in which these organisms are present (all of the industrialized countries of the world) have been responsible for the phenomenon, and for the decreasing therapeutic effectiveness of this drug. In this respect, the epidemiology of the typhoidal and nontyphoidal infections due to salmonella are essentially identical. It is quite apparent that experiences with the increasing problem of episomally-mediated resistance to antibiotics among the salmonellae makes it patently clear that this constitutes a major present and future threat to the effective management of disease caused by this group of organisms.

The largest outbreak of typhoid fever recognized in the United States in over three decades occurred in 1973 at the South Dade Migrant Farm Labor Camp in Dade County, Florida; 225 cases occurred within the camp, 5 outside; 184 patients required hospitalization [73]. The index case was thought to be a mentally retarded child, who appeared to have acquired the infection from an asymptomatic carrier of *S. typhi* who lived in a neighboring house. Subsequent contamination of the flawed water supply of the camp from an inadequate sewerage system resulted in widespread dissemination of the disease. This epidemic makes it clear that segments of society living under conditions in which rapid transmission of the typhoid bacillus may occur are exposed to infection when sewage disposal and water supply are improperly controlled. Similar situations exist throughout the United States and over the rest of the world and require only the introduction of the organism for an epidemic to start.

EPIDEMIOLOGY OF NONTYPHOIDAL SALMONELLOSIS

Nontyphoidal salmonellae have been recovered from a wide variety of species, including chicken, duck, turkey, dove, pigeon, buffalo, pig, sheep, cow, dog, cat, rat, mouse, guinea pig, lizard, flea, cockroach, tick, louse, tortoise, whale, seal, parrot, sparrow, and housefly [78]. The most common sources of non-human isolates of these organisms in the United States in recent years are listed in Table 4. That these are important in the epidemiology of human disease is suggested by the data presented in Table 5; these indicate the ten serotypes isolated most frequently from humans and animals from 1963 to 1973. It is evident that these are similar; this suggests that animal reservoirs are important in the transmission of this kind of disease. Studies in which 53% of human infections have been noted to have been related to disease in abattoirs [79] and reports of outbreaks involving unusual serotypes that have produced disease first in animals and then in man [80,81] confirm this.

Perhaps the most important factor involved in the increase in incidence of disease caused by nontyphoidal salmonellae in the United States has been a progressive trend towards mass processing and distribution of food products, particularly those derived from animals among which these organisms are widely distributed [82]. This is in sharp contrast to the epidemiology of ty-

TABLE 4. Source of Non-human Salmonella Isolates for the Years 1968–1971*

Sources	% of Total	
Turkeys	17.6	Foods Consumed by Man = 68.7%
Chickens	16.3	
Swine	9.4	
Cattle	6.8	
Other domestic animals	5.6	
Eggs and egg products	3.1	
Other foods	9.9	
Animal feeds	19.9	
Reptiles	3.7	
Birds	3.1	
Miscellaneous	4.6	
Total	100	

* Compiled from statistics of the Center for Disease Control [56].

TABLE 5. The Ten Most Frequently Isolated Salmonella Serotypes from Human and Non-human Sources in the United States, 1963–1973*

HUMAN			NON-HUMAN		
Serotype	No. Isolates	% of Total	Serotype	No. Isolates	% of Total
S. typhimurium	69,300	28.4	S. typhimurium	12,339	16.7
S. enteritidis	16,813	6.9	S. heidelberg	6,110	8.3
S. newport	16,495	6.8	S. anatum	4,070	5.5
S. heidelberg	16,389	6.7	S. infantis	3,335	4.5
S. infantis	13,585	5.6	S. saint-paul	3,175	4.3
S. saint-paul	9,969	4.1	S. derby	2,799	3.8
S. derby	8,288	3.4	S. montevideo	2,741	3.7
S. thompson	7,120	2.9	S. choleraesuis	1,974	2.7
S. typhi	6,961	2.8	S. thompson	1,927	2.6
S. blockley	5,317	2.2	S. senftenberg	1,970	2.7
Total	170,237	69.7	Total	40,440	54.8
Total (all serotypes) 244,256			Total (all serotypes) 73,848		

* Compiled from statistics of the Center for Disease Control [56].

phoid and paratyphoid, in which pollution of drinking water supplies and human carriers of the bacteria are primarily involved [83]. As indicated in Table 4, poultry, egg and dairy products, beef and pork constitute an important reservoir for dissemination of salmonella. The extent of the problem is emphasized by the data derived from studies of different commercially prepared foods: 41.4% of turkeys examined in California [84] and 50.2% of chickens cultured in Massachusetts [85] yielded salmonellae; 20.8% of 1131 commercial frozen egg whites were contaminated by these organisms [86]. Salmonella were recovered from 9.9% of 7,000 samples of egg powder used in bakeries, egg drinks, and mayonnaise in England [82]. A large outbreak of infection due to *S. newbrunswick* was related to the ingestion of dried milk powder [87]. Twenty-three per cent of fresh and 12.5% of smoked sausage bought in retail shops have been found to contain these organisms [88]. A large epidemic of gastroenteritis due to *S. java* was traced to commercially prepared smoked whitefish [89]. A recent outbreak of disease due to *S. eastbourne* infection, affecting 23 of the United States and 7 provinces of Canada, was traced to contamination of Christmas-wrapped chocolate balls [90]. This large variety of potentially-contaminated foodstuffs, together with technics of cooking at temperatures too low to achieve sterilization and the use of prepared foods that do not require heating, readily explain the progressively increasing problem of nontyphoidal salmonellosis.

The epidemiologic cycles involved in this type of salmonella-induced disease are complicated and difficult to eradicate. This kind of infection is mainly a zoonosis, with the primary cycle in poultry and livestock [59,82,91]. Infection occurs by direct animal-to-animal spread, but also by the use of feeds contaminated with the organisms [92]. A cycle of transmission from animals has been shown to be of greatest importance [82,92]. In addition, it has become recognized that amplification of this process may occur by contamination of other products, such as dried brewer's yeast [93,94] and carmine dye [95], that are usually not thought to be dangerous in this respect. In these instances, complicated commercial machinery used in the production of these seemingly innocuous substances becomes contaminated, and the "innocent bystanders," the yeast, dye, etc., are then involved secondarily [96]. It is thought that similar mechanisms operate in the spread of salmonella to poultry, eggs and meat; a few infected specimens contaminate the abattoir or processing plant, which then becomes the primary source of dissemination of the organisms to food products originally free of them. Because detection and subsequent destruction of healthy animals and fowl excreting salmonellae is unlikely to be economically feasible, it has been suggested that the following indirect means of limiting the proliferation of nontyphoidal salmonellosis be applied [83]: (a) prevention of the initiation of infection in salmonella-free flocks and herds by eliminating the introduction of animals carrying the organisms and the use of contaminated feed; (b) limitation of the spread of the bacteria after they have been introduced; (c) reduction of contamination by intestinal contents during slaughter; (d) refrigeration of slaughtered animals to prevent growth and multiplication of the bacteria; (e) destruction of salmonella by pasteurization or sterilization after processing, (f) cooking at proper temperature, and prevention of contamination after this has been completed.

Studies of the epidemiology of salmonellosis in New York City by Cherubin and his colleagues [58] have led them to take issue with these comments. They have stressed the importance of person-to-person transmission, particularly in infections caused by *S. typhimurium,* and especially in young children and in groups living in poor socioeconomic situations, for whom effective sanitary control of the environment is essentially lacking. However, a review of their own experiences with this problem in the rest of the United States by the Center for Disease Control [59] has indicated that, although person-to-person transmission represents a potentially important mechanism whereby amplification of the infection within populations may occur, the basic and more important source is contaminated foodstuffs. Thus, it appears that, at present, a significant reduction in the incidence of human salmonellosis will probably be best achieved only by control of contamination and infection of animals and at sites of processing and packing. The conditions required for initiation of a foodborne outbreak of salmonellosis have been defined by Bowmer [97]. They include (a) a reservoir of the infective agent; (b) contamination of an item of food capable of supporting bacterial growth; (c) sufficient and suitable temperature for bacterial multiplication; (d) ingestion of a large enough number of organisms by susceptible persons.

The cost of food-associated outbreaks of salmonellosis is often very high. For example, a recent small food-borne epidemic in Minnesota in which 125 individuals were affected resulted in a net cost of $28,733; $18,413 of this was for lost wages and productivity [98]. Nationally, approximately 2,000,000 cases of this kind of disease occurs in the United States each year; the economic impact of this has been estimated to be 20–200 million dollars. In addition, great expense is often incurred when commercial items found to be contaminated with salmonella are recalled. For example, the cost of recalling salmonella-laden chocolate candy in 1967 was approximately $5,000,000 [2].

The salmonella surveillance program of the Center for Disease Control (CDC) carefully monitors reports of isolations of members of this genus in the United States as a means of detecting epidemics [56,99]. An outbreak is usually recognized when one of the following conditions is present: (a) a rare serotype is identified, (b) an unusually large number of isolations of the same serotype are reported from a defined area, and (c) changes in the normal geographic distribution of certain serotypes are noted. An example of this is the following: While only 3.2% of all the salmonella isolated in the United States in 1967 came from Hawaii, 97% of the organisms recovered in this state were *S. oslo*. The appearance of this species in other parts of the country would then suggest the possibility of an epidemic occurrence, perhaps related to food grown, processed in or shipped from Hawaii. A rapid increase in the presence of a serotype already present in an area, or the introduction of a new one in significant numbers may herald the prospect of an epidemic of salmonellosis caused by that strain [2,99,100]. Two recent international outbreaks of infection due to salmonella emphasize the importance of these epidemiologic principles. Beginning in 1969 and for the next several years, disease caused by *S. agona* became a significant public health problem in the United States, United Kingdom, the Netherlands and Israel. By 1972, it was the eighth most commonly isolated serotype in the United States, and second most common one in the United Kingdom. Epidemiologic investigation starting with study of a small outbreak in Paragould, Arkansas revealed that chicken served in a restaurant in that town had come from a Mississippi poultry farm that fed its birds with feed supplemented with Peruvian fishmeal, a product known to be frequently contaminated by this serotype of salmonella. The use of this animal food in other areas of the world led to an international epidemic that was recognized because of the unusual occurrence of a rare serotype in widely disparate places outside of its usual geographic niche. Although animal feeds contain only 2–10% fishmeal, it was suggested that amplification of the problem of salmonellosis occurred in the following manner: low levels of salmonella in the feed led to asymptomatic infections that were not detected by the usual technics of culture at abattoirs; the commonly-employed methods of processing large numbers of animals in small areas prior to slaughter led to a significant degree of animal-to-animal transmission; asymptomatic carriers, under the stress of transport and processing, excrete an increased number of organisms, with resulting secondary contamination of other animals directly or through infected processing equipment [59,101].

S. eastbourne, previously a rare cause of human infection, was responsible for 80 cases of infection in 23 states of the United States, and for 39 cases in 7 provinces of Canada between December 1973 and February 1974. Epidemiologic study identified Christmas-wrapped chocolate balls made by one manufacturer as the common vehicle. Microbiologic investigation at the factory where the food was made led to definition of cocoa beans as the probable source. The organism was found able to survive the degree of heat usually generated in the process of producing the candy because the moisture content of the chocolate was low. This outbreak was detected because of the unusual number of cases caused by a rare serotype. Subsequent studies of chocolates prepared by other manufacturers disclosed the presence of other more common serotypes than *S. eastbourne*; this finding suggested that this form of candy may be an important source for the dissemination of salmonella over wide geographic areas, especially during holiday seasons when large quantities are sold [90].

In addition to food-borne and person-to-person transmission of nontyphoidal disease due to salmonella in the United States, another source, pet turtles, has been identified and partially controlled. Studies carried out in as widely separated parts of the country as Utah, Connecticut, New Jersey, Georgia (Atlanta), Washington (Seattle) and Minnesota (Minneapolis) have indicated that 9–25% of all instances of salmonellosis in these areas could be traced to contact with these animals. Not surprisingly, the highest incidence was in children who owned pet turtles. The Center for Disease Control has estimated that approximately 280,000 cases of turtle-associated salmonella infection occurred in the United States between 1970 and 1971. The establishment of regulations limiting the sale of these animals offers promise for control of this source of infection [102].

HOSPITAL AND INSTITUTIONAL SALMONELLA INFECTION

Over the thirteen years (since 1963) during which the Center for Disease Control has been involved in nationwide surveillance of the distribution of salmonella in the United States it has become apparent that hospitals, nursing homes, and mental institutions have assumed major importance in the epidemiology of salmonellosis [55,103,104]. Between 1963 and 1972, 112 (28%) of 395 recognized epidemics of this disease occurred in such places; the over-all case-fatality rate of 3,496 cases was 2.3%, considerably higher than the 0.2% reported for noninstitutional outbreaks of this kind of disease. Two groups of patients are at special risk—those in nursing homes and infants in nurseries for the newborn; the incidence of death in these groups has been 8.7 and 7.0%, respectively. In one outbreak in a nursing home, 38% of 104 patients died; in an epidemic involving two pediatric hospitals in Puerto Rico, 14% of the children succumbed to the infection. Three epidemic patterns have been identified when salmonellosis has occurred in institutions. One is related to a common vehicle that has involved primarily adults and frequently more than one hospital; the commonest source of the organisms has been contaminated eggs and egg products. A second is featured by small, but continuing epidemics in nurseries for newborns, pediatric wards and mental institutions, in which cross-infection results from person-to-person spread. The third pattern is characterized by relatively small, repeated or continuing outbreaks due to intermittent consumption, usually by adults, of contaminated but infrequently utilized common vehicles, such as medications, diagnostic agents, etc. These last two types have similar epidemic curves [55,103–105].

The question of the relative importance of exposure to a common source vs. transmission from person-to-person in the institutional setting has received a great deal of attention in the past few years. MacGregor and Reinhart [106] have studied the impact of the admission of eight patients with undiagnosed gastroenteritis due to salmonella to a hospital. Two hundred and sixty-five patients and members of the staff were exposed to the infected individuals. No instances of symptomatic or asymptomatic infection developed in the contacts, despite the lack of efforts to exercise "enteric precautions" in the care of the persons with salmonellosis. This experience led to the conclusion that person-to-person transmission is of little importance in the epidemiology of institutional outbreaks of this kind of infection. However, other investigators have demonstrated that at least five common serotypes of nontyphoidal salmonella are able to persist in appreciable numbers for at least 3 hours on the hands of individuals when inocula as small as 500 organisms have been used [107]. It appears, therefore, that person-to-person transmission may occur, particularly via contamination of the hands. This is probably of most importance in nurseries for the newborn, pediatric hospitals, nursing homes, and facilities for the care of the mentally ill, in which fecal contamination and/or inadequate personal hygiene may be common. A more common situation is that experienced in a hospital in Maine [108] in which 18 individuals developed salmonellosis after ingestion of contaminated eggnog. Fourteen persons among the patients and staff who had contact with the index cases but did not partake of the contaminated food were infected [108]. This again illustrates the extent to which an epidemic of disease caused by salmonella may be amplified to a degree greater than that directly related to ingestion of a contaminated food. The authors of this report, in commenting upon the high rate of person-to-person transmission in some but not all outbreaks of salmonellosis in institutions, suggested the following possible explanations: some serotypes of salmonella, especially *S. heidelberg, S. derby,* and *S. typhimurium,* may be associated with person-to-person transmission more often than other serotypes; larger numbers of highly susceptible patients may be present in some institutions; some hospitals may carry out "enteric precautions" less effectively than others. A recent report of an epidemic of salmonellosis in the pediatric wards of two adjacent hospitals underscores these points [105]. The causative agent was *S. heidelberg,* one of the serotypes associated with a high rate of spread from one individual to another; person-to-person transmission occurred among the patients and staff, and prolonged the outbreak for approximately four months; those in the youngest age group were the most susceptible; institution of cohort-nursing technics and isolation of all patients excreting the organism was necessary to halt the epidemic.

The usual cause of initial cases of nosocomial salmonellosis is a food or medical product ingested either inside or outside the hospital. This may, in turn, be disseminated from one person to another. A particularly notorious example of this phenomenon is a "common source" epidemic of infection due to *Salmonella derby* that occurred in 1963. This was related to eating raw or undercooked eggs that had been distributed widely over the eastern United States and were contaminated by this organism. Epidemiologic investigation revealed 822 cases of salmonellosis caused by this serotype in 53 hospitals in 13 states [109]. Experience with this epidemic led to establishment of a rule, now widely applied in hospitals, that requires all eggs or egg-products to be well-cooked before they are served to patients. Unusual common sources that have been involved in outbreaks of salmonella in hospitals include dried coconut, yeast, carmine dye, and pharmaceutical products of animal origin such as pancreatin, pepsin, bile salts, gelatin, vitamins, and extracts of thyroid gland, adrenal cortex, pancreas, pituitary gland, liver, and stomach [103,104]. Among environmental factors that have been implicated in cross-infections by salmonella are air, dust, respirators in delivery rooms, bedside tables and cribs, thermometers in wooden holders, a thermostatically controlled water bath used to warm baby food, and a sigmoidoscope [110]. A prolonged epidemic of disease caused by *S. choleraesuis* in immunologically compromised patients was traced to transfusion of platelets obtained from a single asymptomatic hematogenous carrier of the organism; this is the first such instance on record [111]. *S. oslo* has recently been reported to have been the cause of a cluster of cases of infection related to the use of an inadequately cleaned fiberoptic endoscope contaminated by the organism. Because of the difficulty of cleaning such fragile and expensive instruments, it may be anticipated that they will probably be involved, as a common source, in other outbreaks of salmonellosis and other infections [112].

In addition to the exposure to an infected common source, as described above, another mechanism by which nosocomial salmonellosis may be initiated is admission to a medical institution of an unsuspected excretor of salmonella.

It is quite common in epidemics in nurseries, for example, for the index case to have been delivered from a mother with undiagnosed diarrhea caused by salmonella. With adults, the asymptomatic carriers may be a special problem, especially if they reside in nursing homes and custodial institutions for the mentally ill and mentally defective [104].

Nosocomial salmonellosis is a continuing and important problem among elderly and very young populations. Because of the relative frequency with which various serotypes of salmonella are circulated within the hospital environment, reports of an unusual propensity to infection associated with a particular underlying disease must be viewed critically. This may be merely a function of the length of time patients and other individuals spend in medical institutions and, by virtue of this, increase the risks of exposure to infection.

CHAPTER III

Pathology and Pathophysiology of Salmonella Infection

Four factors are involved in the pathogenesis of infections caused by salmonella. They are (a) the risk of direct or indirect contact with a particular serotype of the organism, (b) the number of viable bacterial cells ingested, (c) the level of susceptibility of an exposed individual and (d) the characteristics of the salmonella serotype [113]. The problem of risk of contact has been discussed in Chapter II; the role played by the other factors is detailed below.

Events following Salmonella Ingestion

There is a paucity of information concerning the size of the inoculum involved in naturally-acquired disease due to salmonella. Most of what is known has been acquired from studies in volunteers to whom a varying number of organisms have been fed, and from a few carefully investigated common source outbreaks. McCullough and Eisele [114–117] have administered strains of salmonella isolated from purchased samples of spray-dried powdered whole egg to healthy volunteers. Approximately 10^6–10^9 organisms were required to produce disease in more than 50% of these individuals. The specific number of bacteria that constituted an ID_{50} varied with different serotypes of the organism. The rare human pathogen *S. pullorum,* which is highly adapted to chickens, produced infection only when $>10^9$ cells were inoculated; in contrast, *S. newport,* a common cause of disease in man, required only 10^5–10^6 bacteria. Inocula of greater numbers were needed to produce infection in volunteers rechallenged after initial exposure to the same serotype. Smaller numbers of salmonellae dispersed in other foods appear to have been sufficient to produce significant disease in epidemic situations in which less healthy and more susceptible persons and more virulent serotypes were involved [2]. A dessert prepared with contaminated frozen egg yolk containing $<10^2$ *S. typhimurium* per gm has been the cause of a series of outbreaks of food poisoning [56]. As few as 15,000 *S. cubana* per gram of carmine dye given to patients for diagnostic purposes has been responsible for a hospital-associated outbreak of infections, some instances of which terminated fatally [95,96]. Infants fed cereal contaminated with small numbers of *S. muenchen* (7 to 14 organisms per gram) also developed severe salmonellosis [118]. Thus, studies in healthy volunteers involving only a few serotypes and a limited variety of foods may yield results that are not transposable to the usual clinical and epidemiologic experiences with naturally occurring infection in a community [2].

Hornick et al. [23] infected healthy volunteers with the Quailes strain of *S. typhi*; this was isolated from a carrier and contains Vi antigen. None of the individuals became ill when inoculated with 10^3 organisms; of those given 10^5, 10^7 and 10^9 bacteria, 25, 50 and 95%, respectively, developed disease; clinical manifestations did not vary with the size of the inoculum. However, the length of the incubation periods was greater in those receiving smaller inocula. Whether other strains of *S. typhi,* older or younger age, or the use of different types of food as vehicles for the organisms would measurably alter this experience is not clear.

Following ingestion of salmonella, the organisms pass through the stomach into the small bowel before the disease process can be initiated. The bactericidal activity of the normal human stomach produced by the low pH of gastric juice regulates the number of ingested bacteria entering the small intestine [119–123]. Studies of experimental human and animal salmonellosis have indicated that the decrease in acid-content produced by the addition of sodium bicarbonate reduces the size of the inoculum required to cause disease, and that, in this situation, a large number of viable organisms persist in the stomach and bowel [124,125]. A high incidence of salmonellosis has been observed in individuals with surgically induced or other types of achlorhydria (pernicious anemia or atrophic gastritis) [126–129]. Waddell and Kunz [126] postulated that, in addition to the absence of acid in these cases, rapid transit time from stomach to intestine and secondary changes in intestinal flora may play a role in the pathogenesis of the infection. The severity of the disease produced by salmonella in these patients appears to be directly related to the degree of achlorhydria [130–132].

That the medium in which an inoculum of salmonella is ingested may be of some importance is suggested by the evidence recorded above and by a recent experience with a waterborne epidemic of *Salmonella typhimurium* that involved about 16,000 persons [133]. The water incriminated in this outbreak was found to contain 10^3 organisms/liter, an inoculum considerably smaller than that usually considered necessary to produce disease. Despite this, the epidemic was widespread. It was suggested that the reason for this was that water, unlike food, passes rapidly through the stomach and hence organisms which it contains are not subjected to the bactericidal effects of gastric acid. It is clear from such studies that, although the stomach is an effective barrier to the acquisition of salmonellosis, this may be rendered ineffective by large inocula, achlorohydria, rapid gastric transit time, administration of acid buffering agents and protection of the bacteria by the medium in which they are ingested.

The course of events that develops after passage of the salmonella through the gastric barrier depends on multiple factors, the most important of which is probably the serotype of the organism. When *S. typhi* in sufficient quantities is ingested, bacterial multiplication takes place in the intestinal tract during the first four or five days. Penetration of the gut mucosa occurs some time after the initiation of growth of the organism. In addition, there appears to be rapid penetration of the bacilli into the intracellular environment without a period of intraluminal multiplication in a few individuals [23]. The intestinal phase of the disease in man is associated with rather subtle degenerative and proliferative changes in the villi, crypt glands and lamina propria of the upper portion of the small bowel; there is a mononuclear, sometimes granulomatous, reaction in the lamina propria. These changes are unassociated with clinical symptoms and resolve promptly when recovery from disease takes place [134]. Although the infiltrate is composed of mononuclear cells when *S. typhi* is involved, it contains primarily polymorphonuclear leukocytes when other salmonellae produce infection. It has been suggested that differences in phagocytic effectiveness of these two types of inflammatory cells may explain the high incidence of bacteremia with *S. typhi* and the low frequency of this event following invasion by other salmonellae [135,136].

Penetration of the intestinal mucosa is thought to occur primarily in the distal ileum and, perhaps, the cecum and proximal large bowel [137,138]. The exact mechanisms involved in penetration and the subsequent pathogenetic events have, for obvious reasons, not been possible to study in man. Experience with laboratory infection strongly suggests that mucosal invasion occurs through the brush border of the epithelial cell or through intercellular junctional complexes [139,140]. The organisms attach preferentially to the tips of the villi, where they invade and multiply. Only a few villi (< 5% of the total) are involved in the process. This raises the question of whether bacterial attachment is to specific receptor sites or if it occurs in random fashion. There is no evidence of cellular damage or inflammation at the sites of microbial invasion initially. Later, possibly as a result of the activity of chemotactic factors elaborated by the organisms, inflammatory cells appear; these may cause mucosal damage [141,142]. The areas of the intestine first involved are rapidly cleared of salmonella. Meanwhile, the organisms reach and multiply within the intestinal lymph follicles, from which they spread to the draining mesenteric lymph nodes. Studies in a murine typhoid model [138] have demonstrated the preeminence of the distal ileum as the site of penetration by the bacteria; only the lymph nodes draining the ileum were infected with salmonellae in the first 24 hours following intestinal penetration and proliferation. The bacilli spill into the thoracic lymph from the lymph nodes and reach the systemic circulation. There is marked hyperplasia and hypertrophy of all the elements of the reticuloendothelial system (RES) during the period when the organisms are growing in lymphoid tissue. Invasion of the liver (granulomas containing monocytes are present), spleen, gall bladder and bile may take place during the bacteremic phase. Secondary infection of the intestine occurs when bacteria-containing bile reaches it [23,137,141]. The organisms may penetrate distant areas such as bone, meninges, serosal surfaces, soft tissues, etc., during the period of bacteremia.

The course of events that follows ingestion of other species of salmonella depends on the specific serotype involved. Although the pathogenetic processes that occur when *S. paratyphi* A, *S. paratyphi* B (*S. schottmulleri*) or *S. paratyphi* C (*S. hirschfeldi*) are the causative agents have not been examined in great detail, it appears that they are not very different from those initiated by infection with *S. typhi*. Disease caused by *S. anatum* is usually restricted to the intestinal phase; invasion of lymphoid tissue is only occasional, and invasion of the bloodstream is rare. *S. typhimurium* is of intermediate virulence. It may cause symptomatic or asymptomatic intestinal proliferation and, on occasion, enter the blood, but rarely produces the complete clinical syndrome of typhoid fever. The pathogenesis of disease caused by *S. choleraesuis* is unique in that only minimal involvement of the intestine, but rapid and very frequent invasion of the blood, occurs [24]. Kent et al. [143] have developed a guinea pig model for determining virulence of salmonella that makes it possible to predict the series of events most likely to follow infection by different serotypes of the organisms as well as different strains of a specific serotype.

Pathology of Salmonella Infection

The pathologic hallmarks of salmonella infection are reticuloendothelial hyperplasia and hypertrophy of the reticuloendothelial tissues, particularly of the intestinal and abdominal lymph nodes, but also of the spleen, liver, and bone marrow. The basic histologic lesion is an intense phagocytosis of bacteria, senescent white cells and erythrocytes by the activated invading macrophages. Erythrophagocytosis is an unusually prominent microscopic feature characteristic of significant degrees of disease caused by salmonella, especially the enteric fevers. As seen in Figures 3 and 4, small aggregates of reticulum cells and macrophages are present; individual cells are round or oval in shape and possess abundant cytoplasm that contains the products of their phagocytosis [144–148].

When infection due to salmonella is restricted to the intestine (salmonella gastroenteritis), the anatomic abnormalities are most striking in the ileum; involvement of neighboring small bowel and colon is less marked. The inflammatory response is relatively superficial, and is characterized by edema, hyperemia, and diffuse infiltration of the mucosa and lamina propria by

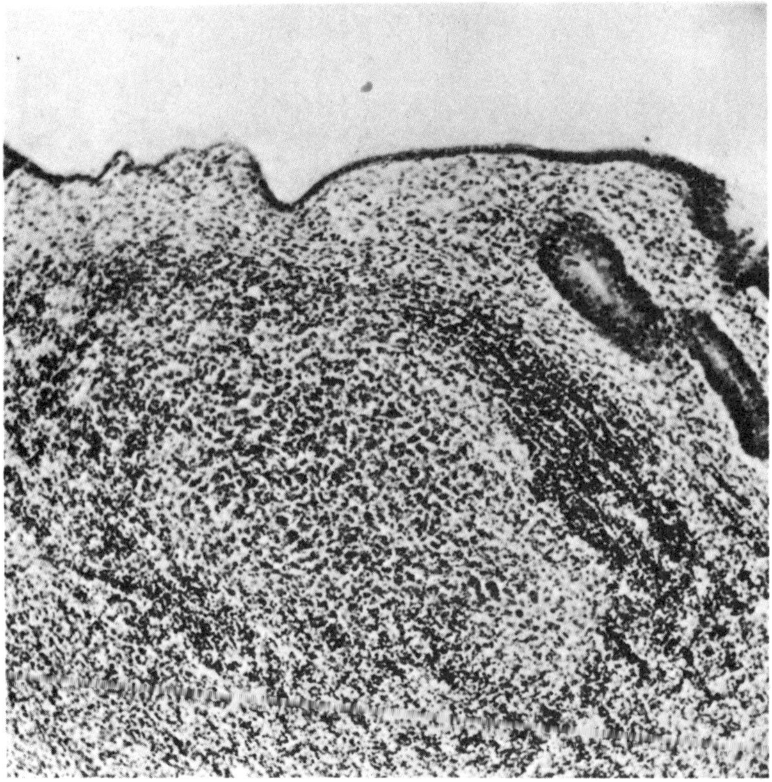

FIG. 3. Low power light microscopic view of a hyperplastic lymphoid follicle in the ileum of a patient with typhoid fever. (From Mallory FB: *The Principles of Pathologic Histology*. WB Saunders, Philadelphia, 1914, p. 164 [145].)

leukocytes. The lymphoid tissue of the bowel and the draining mesenteric lymph nodes are moderately swollen, and may be the site of minute areas of focal necrosis. Splenic hyperplasia of mild-moderate degree is common, but the liver and bone marrow are usually not involved. Ulceration and/or perforation of the intestine is quite uncommon [146].

The sequential changes that occur in the course of severe typhoid fever, particularly those in the gastrointestinal tract, are in sharp contrast to the mild ones described above. Osler [144], Mallory [145] and other students of typhoid fever in the early twentieth century classified the pathologic alterations in the gastrointestinal tract into four stages—*hyperplasia, necrosis and sloughing, ulceration,* and *healing*. The hyperplastic changes begin to appear in the intestinal lymphoid tissue during the first week of clinical illness, and involve primarily the Peyer's patches of the ileum and the solitary lymphoid follicles of the cecum.

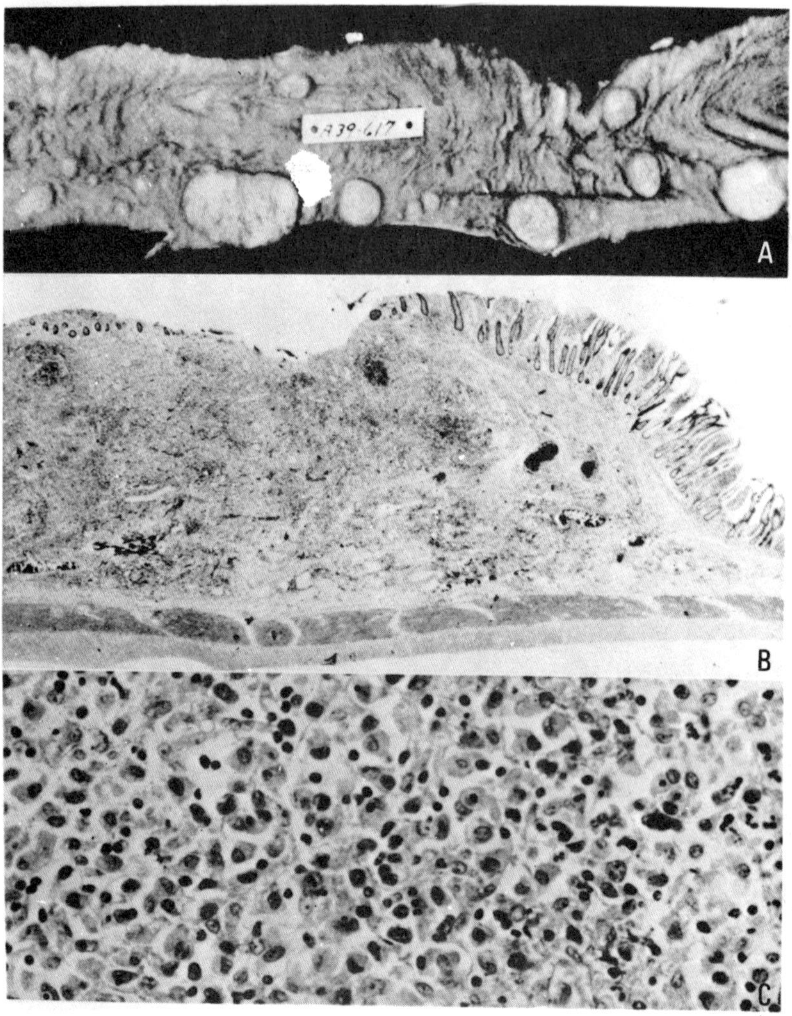

FIG. 4. The ileum in typhoid fever. A. Gross appearance of the markedly hyperplastic lymphoid follicles on the mucosal surface of the ileum. B. Low power light microscopic view of the hyperplastic ileal lymphoid follicle demonstrating necrosis of the overlying bowel mucosa. C. High power light microscopic view of the hyperplastic lymphoid follicle, demonstrating the small aggregates of reticulum cells and macrophages, several of which contain phagocytized erythrocytes and leukocytes. (From Robbins SL: *Textbook of Pathology*. Third Edition. WB Saunders, Philadelphia, 1967, p. 320, 321 [147].)

The follicles are swollen, grayish-white and the patches may project 3 to 5 mm, or may be still more prominent. The solitary glands, which range in size from a pin's head to a pea, are usually deeply inbedded in the submucosa, but project to a variable extent. Occasionally, they are very prominent and may be almost pedunculated. Microscopic examination shows at the onset a condition of hyperaemia of the follicles. Later, there is a great increase and accumulation of cells of the lymph-tissue which may even infiltrate the adjacent mucosa and the muscularis; and the blood-vessels are more or less compressed, which gives the whitish, anemic appearance to the follicles. The cells have all the characters of ordinary lymph-corpuscles. Some of them, however, are larger, epithelioid, and contain several nuclei. Occasionally cells containing red blood-corpuscles are seen. This so-called medullary infiltration, which is always more intense toward the lower end of the ileum, reaches its height from the eighth to the tenth day and then undergoes one of two changes, *resolution* or *necrosis* [*144*] (Fig. *3,4*).

In addition to the microscopic features described by Osler, scattered lymphocytes and plasma cells are present in and around the lesions. Unlike most other forms of acute infection, there is an almost complete absence of polymorphonuclear leukocytes. Mesenteric lymph nodes (particularly those draining the ileum) exhibit hyperplastic changes simultaneously with those in the lymphoid tissue in the wall of the bowel. The sinusoids of the lymph nodes are engorged and distended by large collections of macrophages and reticuloendothelial cells, become swollen and soft, and often contain focal areas of necrosis and hemorrhage (Fig. 5). The types of cells present within the lymph nodes are identical to those infiltrating the lymphoid tissue of the intestinal mucosa. *S. typhi* can usually be recovered, in pure culture, from these areas [144–148].

If the hyperplasia of the lymphoid follicles of the bowel does not resolve, necrosis of the intestinal mucosa develops, usually by the end of the first 7–10 days of clinical illness, probably because the intense lymphoid reaction

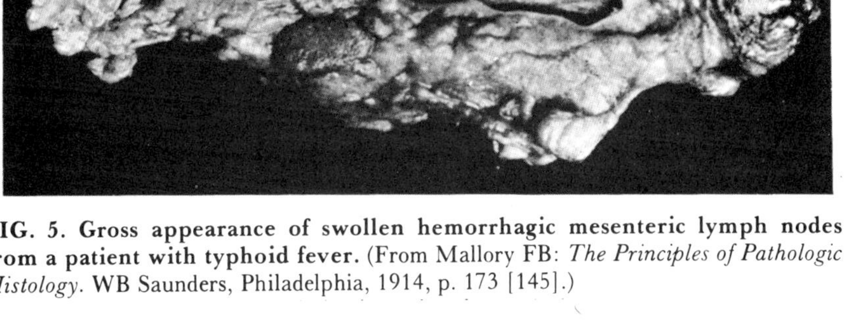

FIG. 5. Gross appearance of swollen hemorrhagic mesenteric lymph nodes from a patient with typhoid fever. (From Mallory FB: *The Principles of Pathologic Histology*. WB Saunders, Philadelphia, 1914, p. 173 [145].)

interferes with the circulation. Sloughing of the overlying mucosa follows and results in the development of an ulcer that may bleed (Figs. 4, 6). The ulcerated lesions are round or oval, and run parallel to the long axis of the bowel, conforming in shape and distribution to the location of the submucosal collections of lymphoid tissue; they are largest in the ileum, the area of the highest concentration of follicles (Figs. 4, 6). The lesions are smaller and more punctate in the cecum and colon, sites in which aggregates of lymphoid cells are not as large as in the ileum. Many of the ulcers are superficial, others penetrate below the submucosa, through the muscular layer and reach the serosa, while still others perforate the entire wall of the intestine and empty into the peritoneal cavity. Their size and number are unrelated to the virulence of the organisms, the degree of bacteremia or the severity of the clinical manifestations. Healing of ulcerated lesions occurs readily, with little or no scarring; simple epithelium free of glands constitutes the cover for these areas. Stricture and obstruction do not complicate healed typhoid fever [144–148].

The spleen is almost invariably enlarged in patients with typhoid fever; it frequently weighs 500–1000 grams. It is cherry-red in color, swollen, tense, quite soft and easily ruptured when handled. Spontaneous rupture during life is quite rare. The most striking microscopic abnormality is the overcrowding of the splenic pulp with enormous numbers of red blood cells, due to both hyperemia and sequestration within the spleen. There is marked reticuloendothelial cellular proliferation and hypertrophy of the splenic sinuses and follicles. The aggregates of these cells form the typical "typhoid nodules"; the individual cells, similar to these in the lymph nodes, exhibit active phagocytosis [144–148].

"Typhoid nodules" are also present in the liver and bone marrow. The liver may be grossly enlarged and swollen. Marked hypertrophy and hyperplasia of the Kupfer cells produces the "nodules." Focal necrosis of nests of hepatocytes is a common feature; the mechanism responsible for this is unknown. It has been suggested that proliferation of Kupfer cells, by producing occlusion of the vascular sinusoids, may cut off blood supply to the cells and lead to their death. Areas of necrosis may appear at any site in the hepatic lobule.

Other organs are less regularly involved during the clinical course of typhoid fever. Swelling and "albuminous" degeneration of the epithelial cells of the proximal tubule of the kidney has been described [144–148]. Focal metastatic areas of pyelonephritis may be present. It has been noted recently that immune complex-induced glomerulonephritis may be a frequent complication of infection by *S. typhi* [149]. The heart is often enlarged. Histologic examination reveals nonspecific patterns of necrosis, degeneration and fatty infiltration of the myocardial cells. The lungs, particularly in the early stages of infection, are the site of bronchitis; pneumonia (possibly of nosocomial origin) may be present late in the disease. Deep venous thrombophlebitis, involving especially the lower extremities and the cerebral venous sinuses, is not uncommon.

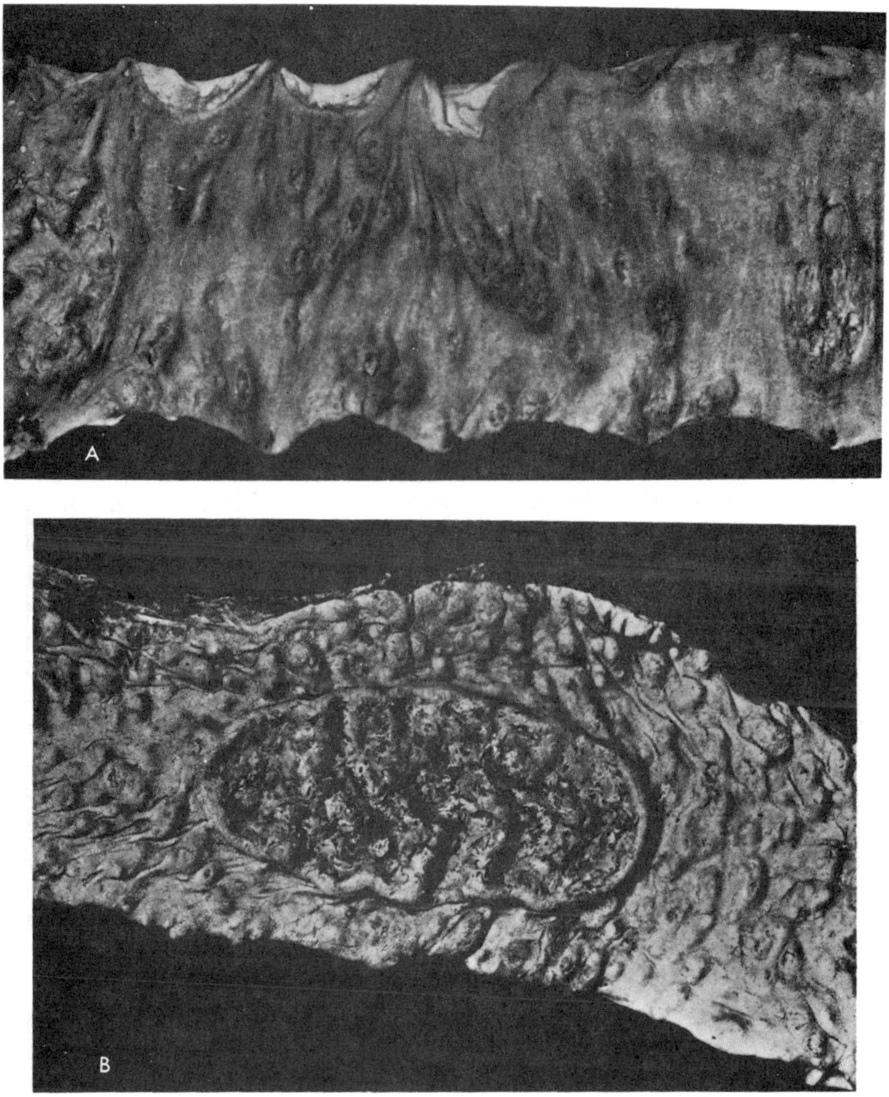

FIG. 6. Gross appearance of the intestine in typhoid fever. A. Affected bowel demonstrating multiple areas of mucosal slough and ulceration. B. Affected bowel demonstrating multiple small areas and a large oval area of mucosal slough running parallel to the long axis of the intestine, and overlying a large hyperplastic lymphoid follicle. (From Mallory FB: *The Principles of Pathologic Histology*. WB Saunders, Philadelphia, 1914, pp. 167, 171. [145].)

Zenker's degeneration may be present in skeletal muscle; this lesion is characterized by loss of transverse striations and swelling and hyalinization of the fibers. The major muscles involved are the rectus abdominis, diaphragm and thigh muscles; rupture and hemorrhage may occur, but are uncommon. Metastatic infections of any organ or tissue, but particularly bone, may develop. These may become manifest during the acute stage of typhoid fever, or lie dormant for months to years. For reasons not clearly understood, metastatic infections caused by *S. typhi,* unlike other lesions produced by this organism, contain polymorphonuclear leukocytes and purulent exudate [144–148].

Mechanisms of Diarrhea Production

The mechanisms involved in the production of the diarrhea that is a common feature of salmonella infection in man and animals has been intensively investigated. Unlike cholera or disease due to enterotoxin-producing strains of *E. coli,* enterotoxin plays no demonstrable role [142]. Mucosal destruction, as is the case in shigellosis, appears not to be of central importance [134–142]. The nature of the interaction between the organisms and the intestinal epithelium appears to be the critical factor. The results of studies of the effects of a number of different strains of *S. typhimurium* on ligated rabbit ileal loop have suggested the following [142]: Only those strains that penetrate the intestinal mucosa are associated with the appearance of inflammatory cells or the elaboration of fluid; noninvasive ones that proliferate in the intestinal lumen but do not invade do not produce these effects. Some strains fail to evoke an inflammatory response, but stimulate secretion of fluid. There appears to be little correlation between the quantity of fluid secreted and the intensity of mucosal inflammation, the number of intramural salmonellae, or the ability of the bacteria to disseminate from the ileum into the bloodstream. This dissociation between initiation of the secretion of fluid and access to the circulation may explain the clinical observation that *S. choleraesuis* rarely produces gastrointestinal symptoms, but is commonly featured by bacteremia. Results of these studies suggest that, once mucosal invasion has occurred, some additional bacterial factor or property is required for the initiation of increased fluid production and diarrhea.

The nature of the alterations in transport of salts and water responsible for the diarrhea of salmonella infection has received a great deal of attention. Powell et al. [150–152] have demonstrated a marked increase in secretion of water, sodium, potassium and chloride ions, and absorption of bicarbonate in the ileum of rats; uninfected animals exhibited an exactly opposite pattern. *In vitro* studies of rabbit ileal mucosa infected with *S. typhimurium* have indicated inhibition of active sodium absorption, without interference with glucose-facilitated sodium absorption. This explains the clinical effectiveness of glucose-containing electrolyte solutions in repleting the deficiency of sodium in patients with diarrhea due to salmonellosis. Active secretion of chloride is stimulated [153]. Transport of water appears to follow the changes in handling of sodium and chloride, and causes the diarrhea. The diarrheal fluid is rich in both protein and potassium. This is thought to reflect local destruction of tissue and release of protein and potassium from cells into the lumen of the intestine. Studies using radioactively labeled mannitol and albumin have failed to generate any evidence that excessive plasma filtration or leakage caused by the inflammatory reaction or invasion of tissue by salmonella play an important role in the pathogenesis of the diarrhea [154]. Investigation of the effects of infection of intact Rhesus monkeys with salmonella, a model thought to most closely approximate human disease, has shown that jejunal, ileal, and colonic dysfunction are of importance in the pathogenesis of the diarrhea [155]. While bacterial invasion and the resulting inflammation of the ileum and colon were found to be associated with changes in transport of salt and water in these areas, abnormalities of jejunal function were not related to invasion or striking morphologic changes.

A critical matter is the nature of the mechanisms involved in altering transport of salts and water if this is not produced by an enterotoxin. Because theophylline, an inhibitor of the phosphodiesterase that normally breaks down cyclic AMP, has been noted to duplicate the changes in transport associated with the diarrhea produced by salmonella [153], and because cyclic AMP alone [156] and cholera enterotoxin, acting through the induction of adenylate cyclase and the elaboration of cyclic AMP [157], produce similar abnormalities in transport, attention has been turned to the adenylate cyclase cyclic AMP system in the intestine as the mechanism possibly involved in the pathogenesis of the diarrhea caused by salmonella. An elegant set of experiments carried out by Gianella and his colleagues have revealed the following series of biochemical events [158,159]: A strain of *S. typhimurium* that invaded the intestinal mucosa and induced fluid secretion caused an increase in the activity of adenylate cyclase and in the concentration of cyclic AMP. Another strain of the organism that was invasive but did not stimulate the secretion of fluid had no effect on either adenylate-cyclase or cyclic AMP. In contrast, the activity of phosphodiesterase, Na-, K- and Mg-ATPase remained normal despite infection with diarrhea-producing organisms. Pretreatment of the animals with indomethacin, a potent inhibitor of the synthesis of prostaglandins, blocked both diarrhea and the associated increase in the activity of adenylate cyclase and cyclic AMP. Previous studies had indicated that prostaglandins increase cyclic AMP by stimulating the activity of adenylate cyclase [159–161]. Presently available data appear to indicate that the diarrhea induced by infection by salmonella is caused by the initiation of synthesis of specific prostaglandins in the intestine. This raises the possibility that anti-prostaglandins may be of value in the management of salmonella-associated diarrhea.

The critical events leading to infection by salmonella are currently thought to be as follows (Fig. 7): (a) Delivery of a sufficient number of pathogenic organisms to the proximal small bowel, followed by intraluminal proliferation; (b) penetration of the ileum and, to a lesser extent, the colon by the invading bacteria and establishment of an inflammatory reaction; (c) stimulation of the synthesis of prostaglandins which activate the adenylate cyclase system, resulting in accumulation of cyclic AMP, block of sodium absorption and secretion of chloride ion, the series of phenomena responsible for diarrhea; (d) interaction of the organisms, following mucosal penetration, with local host defense

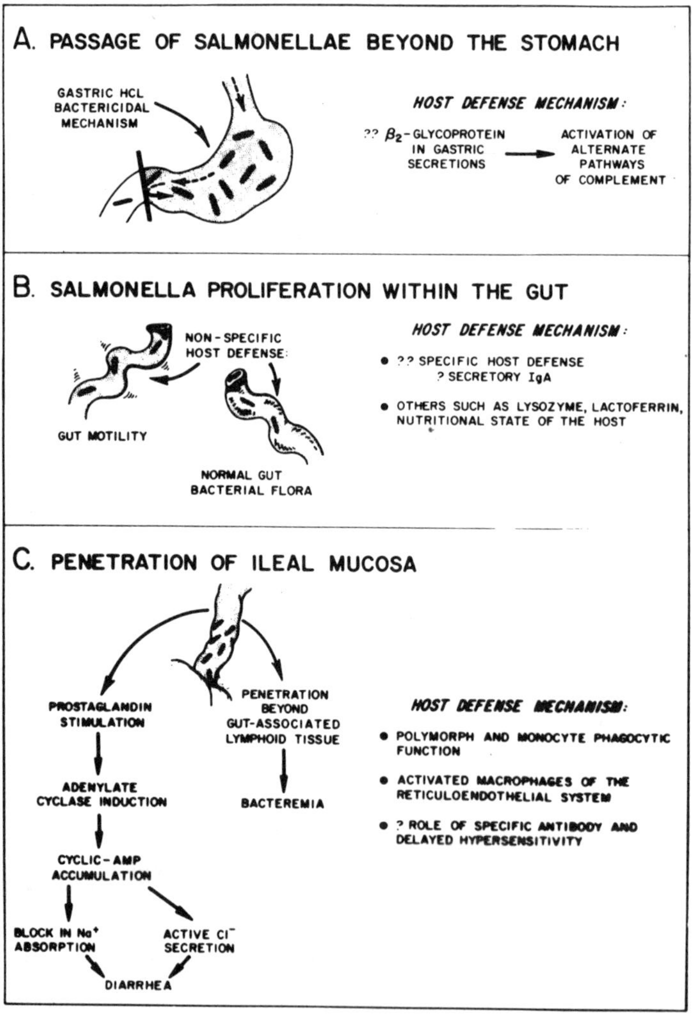

FIG. 7. Schematic representation of the critical steps in the pathogenesis of salmonella infection.

mechanisms, the process that determines access to the regional lymph nodes, thoracic duct and the systemic circulation. These last two events may occur singly or together, or not at all, following invasion of the intestinal mucosa. This determines whether the carrier state, gastroenteritis, and/or symptomatic bacteremia and metastatic infection develops. The interplay between the characteristics of a particular serotype and the activity of both specific and nonspecific host defense mechanisms determines the outcome at each of the critical stages following the initial intrusion of salmonella.

Host Defense against Salmonella Infection

In addition to gastric acid, a variety of *nonspecific* factors that play a role in defense against infection are of importance in determining the outcome of ingestion of salmonella [137] (Fig. 7): these include (a) the physical barrier to epithelial penetration imposed by intestinal mucus, (b) the cleansing effect of intestinal motility on the upper area of the bowel (diarrhea resulting from increased intestinal motility may be considered a protective mechanism; systemic salmonellosis with bacteremia has occasionally followed treatment with opiates in patients with otherwise mild gastroenteritis) [162,163], (c) lysozyme present in the secretions, (d) the bacteriostatic activity of the lactoferrin present in the stomach and gut [164], (e) β_2-glycoprotein of gastric juice, known to act as proactivator in the alternate pathway of activation of complement [164–166], and (f) perhaps the nutritional state of individuals exposed to salmonella. Studies of experimental infection with *S. typhimurium* in rats have indicated that administration of an iron-deficient diet after weaning increased susceptibility to invasion by the organism; the highest rates of morbidity and death were noted in marginally-deficient animals [167,168]. Establishment of iron-deficiency prior to weaning led to persistent decrease in resistance to infection, even when this was later completely corrected. (These observations may be of importance in humans, especially children, who subsist on diets containing marginal or low quantities of iron, as is the case in many of the developing areas in the world.) The mechanism by which nutritional deficiency increases susceptibility of animals to microbial infection may involve a defect in the mobilization of myeloperoxidase-containing leukocytes (iron is an important cofactor for the enzyme) in the lamina propria and submucosa, sites into which salmonella penetrate.

The relative importance of the nonspecific mechanisms of defense discussed above is, for the part, unknown. However, one that appears to play an important role is the normal or autochthonous flora of the intestinal tract. As long ago as 1916, Nissle [169] suggested that this bacterial population was instrumental in preventing the implantation of enteric pathogens in the bowel. Bohnhoff et al. [170], noted that oral administration of streptomycin to mice greatly increased their susceptibility to invasion by *Salmonella enteritidis*; the

ID_{50} was decreased from approximately 10^7 to <10 organisms. They suggested that elimination of gram-negative bacilli, especially *Bacteroides,* from the microflora by the antibiotic was responsible for this phenomenon [171]. The mechanism involved in the protective effect of the normal intestinal flora appears to be, in large part, the production of volatile fatty acids and the associated decrease in oxidation-reduction of the intestinal contents [172–175]. In addition, Wawszkiewicz et al. [176] have described a "Salmonella resistance factor" or *pacifarin* produced by enteric organisms, especially in nutritionally deprived animals, that may be important in preventing implantation of salmonella. The bacteriocins produced by the gram-negative members of the microflora of the gut may interfere with multiplication of salmonella in the intestional tract by such mechanisms as blocking oxidative phosphorylation and inhibiting synthesis of protein. Whether other factors are protective is not known. Nevertheless, it seems clear that the autochthonous microbial flora of the intestinal tract make this area a poor site for the multiplication of salmonella, under normal circumstances. This is emphasized by the established fact that the administration of antibiotics, purgatives or opiates, and surgery involving the bowel, all of which may alter the microbial population qualitatively, quantitatively, or both, increase susceptibility to infection by salmonella.

Study of *specific* factors that determine susceptibility to intestinal infection by salmonella and other enteric pathogens is in its infancy. It has been pointed out that human intestinal tissues, because of the extensive population of plasma cells and lymphocytes in the lamina propria, Peyer's patches, lymphoid follicles of the submucosa, and mesenteric lymph nodes, may constitute the most important immunologic organ of the body [137]. These collections of lymphoid tissue have been shown, in experimental models, to localize and restrict the spread of salmonella [177,178]. The organisms survive and multiply within the macrophages of the reticuloendothelial system (RES) [179,180]. Activation of these cells appears to be responsible for controlling invasion by salmonella, although antibody may play a role in facilitating phagocytosis [181,182]. Phagocytic activity of the RES has been noted to be markedly increased during typhoid fever, especially as a result of heightened activity of the RES in the liver and spleen [183,184]. Once salmonella have penetrated into these cells, they are protected against the effects of humoral antibody and administered antibiotics [185–187]. Miller et al. [188] have noted that phagocytosis of virulent strains of *S. typhi* by nonactivated human leukocytes is not associated with the usual postphagocytic augmentation in oxygen consumption (via the hexose monophosphate pathway), a phenomenon that occurs when gram-positive cocci or avirulent strains of *S. typhi* are phagocytized. That this "defect" in function of leukocytes may be important in the pathogenesis of typhoid fever is suggested by two clinical observations: Sickle cell disease, a disorder associated with a markedly increased risk of severe salmonellosis (Chapter IV), is characterized by a similar deficit in postphagocytic activity of the hexose monophosphate pathway and oxygen consumption [189]. In addition, repeated episodes of systemic disease due to salmonella have been observed in a female heterozygous for chronic granulomatous disease [190]. Cherubin et al. [191] have noted an increased incidence of salmonella bacteremia in children homozygous for this disorder. These observations underscore the great importance of active phagocytic function in the control of the extent and severity of infections caused by salmonella.

Webster [192], as long ago as 1933, reported that resistance to invasion by salmonella in mice was genetically determined, and suggested that it was determined by a simple dominant gene. Gowen later confirmed this observation, but thought that it represented a polygenic mode of inheritance [195]. Recent studies by Plant and Gynn [194,195] have substantiated the importance of genetic determinants in mice. They found that they were not linked to H-2 (histocompatibility determinants in the mouse) or known Ir (immune response) genes, and appeared to correlate with the ability to develop an effective delayed-type hypersensitivity reactions to an extract of *S. typhimurium*; they agreed that susceptibility to salmonellosis is determined in a simple mendelian dominant manner. It has been suggested that cell-mediated immunity is important in the defense against invasive infections caused by salmonella [196].

Allardyce et al. [197] have demonstrated the presence of specific antibodies for *S. typhimurium* in the colostrum of women who have had gastroenteritis due to this organism during pregnancy. This is consistent with the possibility that secretory IgA plays an important role in the defense against invasion by salmonella. Whether production of this globulin, and enhancement of phagocytosis by it—together with mobilization of complement, cell-mediated immunity or circulating humoral antibody play additional roles has not been determined. The fact that the carriage of typhoidal and nontyphoidal salmonella is not associated with clinical manifestations suggests that local intestinal immunity is involved in preventing invasion and infection [137].

Immunity to reinfection is, at best, incomplete in typhoid fever. Relapses occur in approximately 10% of patients who survive without chemotherapy, and in about 20% treated with chloramphenicol [23,63]. The attack rates in two epidemics of typhoid fever occurring five months apart have been noted to be similar [198], even among those involved in the first outbreak. Extensive field trials [199,200] have indicated that most killed typhoid vaccines administered parenterally reduce the incidence of disease in *endemic* areas. Studies of Hornick et al. [23,186] have shown that such preparations are effective in decreasing the incidence of infection only in persons exposed to relatively small numbers of bacteria. This is apparently the situation in nature. The manner in which killed vaccines produce their effect is not clear. There appears to be a very poor correlation between protection against *S. typhi* and circulating antibody to its O, H, or Vi antigens [14,23,137,201,202]. In general, typhoid fever is associated with the development of cell-mediated immunity against the organism, IgM antibodies to its O and H antigens and increases in the level of serum complement [203,204]. Three recent reports [205–207] of salmonellosis in immunosuppressed patients have indicated that both humoral and cellular immunity are important in protecting against this disease. Four of nine individuals with adult "acquired" agammaglobulinemia developed chronic infection; a 10 month old child with high serum IgA, virtually absent IgG and IgM and defective cellular immunity had chronic disease due to *S. blockley* that failed to respond to treatment with gamma globulin or plasma; seven of 146 patients with transplanted kidneys receiving immunosuppressive drugs developed infection of the urinary tract caused by salmonella; 5 had bacteremia. The infectious processes in this group of patients were resistant to specific antimicrobial therapy and persisted for an average of 6.4 months.

In an attempt to explain the high incidence of bacteremia among neonates with gastroenteritis due to salmonella, Rice et al. [105] suggested that the following mechanisms were probably of special importance in conditioning susceptibility to invasion of the bloodstream: (a) chemotaxis for polymorphonuclear leukocytes by serum of newborn children may be defective, the cells appearing to respond sluggishly to normal chemotactic factors; (b) the serum of very young babies is deficient in opsonizing activity, IgM and complement; (c) the response of mononuclear leukocytes to infection is delayed; and (d) there is a relative deficiency of secretory IgA early in life. The combined effects of these immunologic abnormalities make the neonatal child uniquely susceptible to invasion and infection by salmonella.

Metabolic Effects of Salmonella Infection

A number of metabolic studies have been carried out on patients with infections due to salmonella, especially *S. typhi*. Although these have yielded reproducible results in humans and primates with typhoid fever, it appears that most, if not all, of the abnormalities may be present in any infectious process complicated by bacteremia, and are not restricted to typhoidal disease. Some of the metabolic disturbances that have been observed are (a) increase in plasma triglycerides, pre-beta, and alpha-lipoproteins, and (b) decrease in phospholipids, cholesterol and beta-lipoproteins in monkeys infected with *S. typhimurium;* concentrations of free fatty acids have been variable [208]. Human volunteers infected experimentally with *S. typhi* have exhibited a decrease in levels of iron and zinc and an increase in copper in their serum just prior to the onset of clinical manifestations. Small quantities of serum (1 ml) obtained from these patients produced a similar drop in the level of zinc and a flux of amino acids into the liver when injected into rats; this suggests that an endogenous mediator for these effects was liberated into the blood during the early stage of typhoid fever [209,210]. Circulating levels of amino acids, especially alanine, glycine, proline, lysine, and threonine were depressed at the onset of infection;

this was possibly related to their flow into the liver [209,211,212]. Studies of thyroid function in humans and rhesus monkeys infected with salmonella have indicated an increase in the cellular uptake and metabolism of thyroxine (T_4) during the course of disease due to *S. typhimurium, E. coli* and *S. pneumoniae*. This may be related to increased activity of the reticuloendothelial system, a decrease in thyroxine-binding proteins and/or an inhibitor to T_4 binding that develops in response to the infection [213,214]. Although these phenomena represent changes in metabolic homeostasis, their significance in the production of manifestations of disease or in the mobilization of mechanisms of defense is presently not clear.

Effects of Endotoxin

As discussed in Chapter I, salmonellae, like the other *Enterobacteriaciae,* possess a unique lipopolysaccharide constituent, endotoxin, in the cell wall. Many of the clinical manifestations of infection due to these organisms, especially the syndromes of enteric fever, are characterized by phenomena induced by its effects [29]. The best known and well characterized activity of this substance is the production of fever [214]; the pyrogenic reaction is mediated by the following mechanisms; (a) stimulation of polymorphonuclear leukocytes and fixed tissue macrophages to elaborate and release *endogenous pyrogens*; this process requires *de novo* synthesis of protein and RNA; (b) action of the *endogenous pyrogen* on the thermoregulatory center in the anterior hypothalamus [215]. There is also some evidence that endotoxin may, under some circumstances, exert its effect directly upon the thermoregulatory center to produce fever [216]. Multiple exposures to the lipopolysaccharide result in tachyphylaxis, *endotoxin tolerance,* as indicated by decrease in pyrogenicity [29]. Patients with typhoid fever hyper-react to endotoxin on first exposure to it; however, following recovery, they are strikingly tolerant [217,218].

Endotoxin exerts a significant effect upon a variety of plasma peptides that possess important biologic activity. Disseminated intravascular coagulation may be initiated because the lipopolysaccharide (a) induces release of platelet factor 3 and the subsequent generation of thromboplastin through the extrinsic clotting system, or (b) activates Hageman factor (factor XII), an effect that triggers the entire intrinsic "clotting cascade" [219,220]. In addition, both the classic and alternate pathways of complement are activated; this leads to the generation of the mediators of inflammation [221–223]. Pooling of white blood cells, erythrocytes and platelets in the splanchnic and pulmonary vessels follows production of vasoactive substances from these plasma peptides. Depression of myocardial function is induced by endotoxin [224–226]. The sum of these effects is responsible for the development of a syndrome identical to septic shock produced by *intact* bacteria.

Severe leukopenia follows exposure to endotoxin initially, as a result of an increase in margination of circulating granulocytes at the capillary endothelium [227]; this is followed by a marked leukocytosis, due to release of large numbers of cells from the bone marrow [228]. Endotoxin produces aggregation and degranulation of platelets, and increased activity of platelet factor 3 [219,229–232], processes critical in the metabolism of the lipopolysaccharide molecule by the reticuloendothelial system (233).

Endotoxin exerts marked metabolic effects. As a result of its activity on the hypothalamic-pituitary-adrenal axis, it stimulates the elaboration of large amounts of ACTH, cortisol and growth hormone; there is little effect on the other anterior pituitary hormones [234–236]. Exposure to the lipopolysaccharide initially induces hyperglycemia; this is followed by hypoglycemia and depletion of stores of glycogen in the liver as a result of inhibition of gluconeogenesis [237,238]. Abnormalities of lipids, especially an increase in plasma triglycerides and free fatty acids, also develop [29]. Synthesis of protein by the liver is increased [239]. A decrease in serum iron and iron binding capacity and level of zinc in the blood is produced by endotoxin; these phenomena are possibly mediated by endogenous pyrogen [240–244]. Thus, many of the metabolic effects observed in the course of experimental typhoid fever are reproduced by the administration of the lipopolysaccharide.

Endotoxin exerts a profound effect on specific and nonspecific resistance to infection. It is an excellent mitogen for lymphocytes; this may be the reason for its adjuvant effect on the synthesis of antibody [245–247]. However, depending on the nature of the antigen, its dose, and the interval between administration of the antigen and the lipopolysaccharide, an immunosuppressive effect may be produced [248]. After an initial period of increased susceptibility to infection, injection of endotoxin results in an increase in resistance to invasion by bacteria, fungi, viruses and parasites [29]. Multiple factors are responsible for these effects. Among them are increased activity of fixed and circulating phagocytes, and changes in the metabolism of iron and synthesis of antibodies. Whether or not these phenomena play a role in limiting the extent and duration of typhoid fever is presently unknown.

It is clear that salmonellae elaborate significant quantities of endotoxin, and that this interacts with the patient, as evidenced by the shift in reactivity to the lipopolysaccharide from a hyperreactive to a tolerant state during the course of the disease. Many of the effects on metabolism, white blood cells, platelets and serum proteins produced by endotoxin are similar to those present in clinical and experimental infections caused by *S. typhi*.

CHAPTER IV

Clinical Features of Salmonellosis

The clinical manifestations of human salmonellosis can be divided into four syndromes: *gastroenteritis, bacteremia,* with or without focal extraintestinal infection, *enteric fevers* (typhoid-like disease) and asymptomatic *carrier state* [249]. Acute infections of the intestinal tract constitute ⅔ of all recognized disease caused by salmonella [24,63,250,251]. Although this classification is generally useful in practice, it is frequently not possible to sharply delineate each syndrome. For example, gastroenteritis may be complicated by bacteremia and focal lesions, and the carrier state may be a consequence of any of the syndromes [249–251]. It should also be emphasized that every serotype of salmonella has the potential to produce any one of the clinical pictures. Despite this, it is clear that certain ones are consistently associated with specific constellations of manifestations. *S. typhi* and the paratyphoid group of organisms are the causes of enteric fever; *S. newport* and *S. enteritidis* are the primary etiologic agents of gastroenteritis; *S. choleraesuis* is most commonly responsible for bacteremia and focal infection; *S. anatum* usually produces mild gastrointestinal disease and the carrier state. *S. typhimurium* is of particular interest because it is not only the most common species of salmonella involved in the pathogenesis of gastroenteritis, but is also a frequent cause of bacteremia and focal infection. In addition, a number of diseases such as neoplastic disorders, hemoglobinopathies, schistosomiasis, atherosclerosis and inflammatory disease of the bowel, among others, predispose to invasion by specific serotypes of salmonella (249–251).

GASTROENTERITIS

Salmonella are responsible for about 10–15% of all instances of acute gastroenteritis ("food poisoning") that occur in the United States every year [56]. The incubation period of this syndrome averages 8–48 hours; it may be as long as 7 days in experimentally infected volunteers [116]. The initial symptoms are nausea and vomiting. These subside within a few hours, but are followed quickly by abdominal cramps and diarrhea. The pain is typically located in the upper abdomen in the periumbilical area or in the right lower quadrant. Diarrhea persists for 3–4 days and then disappears rapidly. A good diagnostic rule is that diarrhea persisting for longer than a week should be investigated for causes other than salmonella. However, symptoms of infection may be present for 2–3 weeks. The spectrum of manifestations of the gastroenteritis caused by salmonella may be very mild, with a total of one or a few loose stools; to very severe cholera-like with severe abdominal pain, 20–40 loose stools per day leading to dehydration, convulsions and death; or dysentery-like with bloody, slimy stools and marked tenesmus [249,250]. In general, pain in the left lower quadrant, rectal urgency, tenesmus and grossly bloody and purulent stools, the characteristic features of shigellosis, are absent when salmonella is involved. Patients with achlorhydria, particular when it is the result of vagotomy and gastric surgery, appear to be especially susceptible to the cholera-like form of disease [130–132,252].

The temperature is moderately elevated (<102°F) in about 50% of cases, and usually returns to normal within one or two days. High and persistent fever is rarely present; however, when such occurs, bacteremia and/or focal lesions should be suspected. The incidence of transient intrusion of organisms into the blood in uncomplicated gastroenteritis due to salmonella in otherwise healthy adults is about 1 to 4%. This may be an unduly low estimate, due to the infrequency with which properly timed cultures of the blood have been obtained [58]. Infants less than one year of age and adults over the age of 50 generally experience more severe disease and a higher fatality rate.

Physical findings include moderate abdominal tenderness, increased peristalsis and a varying degree of systemic "toxicity." In the more severe forms of the disease, the abdominal signs may mimic those of acute appendicitis, cholecystitis or a ruptured viscus [24,250].

Other than microbiologic studies, the laboratory examinations in this type of infection are relatively nonspecific. The white blood cell count is usually normal; a mild leukocytosis is sometimes present. The sedimentation rate is either normal or slightly elevated; it is high most often when the process is complicated by bacteremia, focal metastatic involvement or perforation of the bowel. Although grossly bloody stools are uncommon in adults, occult fecal blood is detectable intermittently. A very important diagnostic point is the presence of a *moderate* number of polymorphonuclear leukocytes among the mucoid particles of the diarrheal stool. In contrast, the gastroenteritis caused by the enterotoxin of *S. aureus,* endotoxin-producing *E. coli, V. cholerae* and a variety of viral agents is characterized by the absence of neutrophiles. *Many* polymorphonuclear cells, blood and mucous are also present in the fecal discharges of patients with dysentery caused by *Shigella* [162]. Serologic studies (agglutinins for salmonella) are of little diagnostic value. The diagnosis is established by isolation of the organism. Simultaneous infection by more than one serotype occurs occasionally; the clinical manifestations in such cases do not differ from those produced by a single strain [253–256]. (See Illustrative Cases 1, 4, pp. 70, 72.)

Although very few patients with gastroenteritis due to salmonella have had a barium enema during the acute phase of the disease, the following abnormalities have been noted in those who have undergone this procedure [257]: (a) ulceration, edema and dilatation of the duodenum, jejunum and ileum, (b) dilution of barium by excess secretions, (c) diffuse dilatation of the colon, (d) widespread distal colonic edema and superficial ulceration, and (e) segmental distribution of ulcers in the descending colon. Similar abnormalities are present in other inflammatory disorders of the bowel, particularly regional enteritis and ulcerative colitis. A history of prior intestinal disorders, the clinical course, and, most importantly, serial radiologic studies usually serve to distinguish transient abnormalities associated with salmonellosis from those produced by other types of recurrent or persistent disease of the intestine.

The manifestations of gastroenteritis due to salmonella in children frequently differ significantly from those in adults [258–261]. The mean duration of symptoms may be as long as 8.7 days [258]. The severity of the disease tends to be greater and the incidence of bacteremia is probably higher. Grossly bloody stools are common. Cramping pain in the left lower quadrant of the abdomen and tenesmus are frequent features. The effects of the diarrheal loss of fluid and electrolytes may be very profound. Prolonged intestinal carriage of salmonella appears to be a special feature of the disease in infants. However, establishment of a permanent carrier state is quite rare. The potential seriousness of salmonellosis involving the intestine in young children is reflected by the development of chronic diarrhea associated with persistence of the organisms; premature babies may develop necrotizing enterocolitis, the fatality rate of which is very high [259].

Gastroenteritis due to salmonella may present special and occasionally difficult problems for surgeons because it can mimic or complicate other abdominal disorders that ordinarily demand surgical intervention. The two situations in which this is most common are "*salmonella appendicitis*" and postsurgical diarrhea [251]. "*Salmonella appendicitis*" occurs primarily during the first two decades of life [262]. The organisms lodge in the appendix in the course of the gastroenteritis and may produce inflammation or rupture of the organ [263]. Many patients with salmonellosis operated on for appendicitis have normal or mildly inflammed appendices but acute enteritis involving the lower ileum [264–266]. This may be self-limited and not require surgical intervention. A 10 year old boy who was operated on for presumed acute appendicitis but was found to have only enlarged inflamed lymph nodes from which *S. enteritidis* was recovered has been described by Meng [267]; the organism was also present in the feces. Histologic study of the lymphoid tissue revealed hyperplasia; the appendix was normal. It is apparent that salmonella may produce clinical syndromes resembling "appendicitis" but in which all the symptoms are due only to the enteritis, infection of the appendix, mesenteric adenitis without intestinal inflammation, or perforation of the bowel at sites distant to the appendix. It is also clear that unrelated intercurrent appendicitis may appear in the course of invasion of the gut by salmonella. Clinical differentiation of these entities is often very difficult, if not impossible. If there is even the slightest doubt as to the etiology of the abdominal complaints, it is probably best to carry out laparotomy, especially if signs of peritoneal irritation are present. (See illustrative Case 2, p. 71.)

Postoperative disease due to salmonella may present with a variety of syndromes. Infection of the wound or acute cholangitis may be caused by these organisms in patients after cholecystectomy if they are present in the biliary tree [251,268,269]. Fulminant enteritis due to salmonella has been observed after gastrointestinal tract surgery; whether the procedure activates a latent infection or is related to contamination during operation is not known [251,270,271]. Invasion of the bowel by salmonella may follow surgery involving a sterile viscus in patients who are asymptomatic carriers of the organism [251]. The mechanisms involved in this complication are unknown. Among the factors that may play a role, alone or in concert, are disorders of intestinal motility, changes in the microflora of the bowel, hypotension, impaired intestinal circulation and surgical trauma. Surgeons who have removed gallbladders containing *S. typhi* may themselves develop typhoid fever. (See Illustrative Case 3, p. 72.)

Acute gastroenteritis is the most commonly recognized form of human infection caused by salmonella; nontyphoidal serotypes are most often involved (Table 3). Their ubiquity in foodstuffs makes it evident that challenge with varying numbers of different strains and species of these organisms must be common. Both the risk of developing disease and its intensity are dependent on the interaction of the factors discussed in Chapter III. Because acute gastroenteritis caused by nontyphoidal types of salmonella does not appear to induce adequate immunity, repeated episodes of infection, even due to the same serotype, may occur in the same individual [24]. This makes it clear that this syndrome will continue to be an important clinical and public health problem in the foreseeable future.

THE ENTERIC FEVERS

The enteric fevers are characterized by the following features: (a) Prolonged fever, (b) sustained presence of salmonella in the bloodstream without endothelial or endocardial involvement, (c) marked stimulation of the reticuloendothelial system, especially of the intestine and mesentery (the sites first invaded by the organisms) but also of the liver, spleen and nondraining lymph nodes and (d) the development of dysfunction of multiple organs as a result of metastatic spread of the organism, the formation and deposition of immune complexes or the effect of undefined "toxicity."

Although enteric fever may be caused by any serotype of salmonella, the species most often responsible are *S. typhi, S. paratyphi. S. schottmulleri* and *S. hirschfeldi. S. schottmulleri* is presently the commonest nontyphoidal cause of this syndrome in the United States [56]. Regardless of the serotype involved, the pathogenesis and manifestations of enteric fever are qualitatively identical. The severity of the disease, its fatality and relapse rates, the duration, and the incidence and intensity of complications are greater in patients infected by *S. typhi* than in those invaded by other species of salmonella [272]. Since typhoid fever is the prototype of enteric fever and has been studied the most extensively, it is discussed here in greatest detail. Its clinical features may be classified into four stages; (a) those that characterize the incubation period and prodromal stage, (b) those that are present when the active disease has been established, (c) those that result from the development of complications, and (d) those associated with the asymptomatic carrier state.

The length of the incubation period of enteric fever is directly related to the number of organisms to which patients are exposed; the larger the inoculum, the shorter the time between contact and the appearance of illness. This is usually 1 to 2 weeks, but may be as short as 3 or as long as 60 days [23,24]. The greater the number of bacteria ingested, the more severe the manifestations in the incubation period; when only few bacilli are involved, this phase may be entirely asymptomatic. Symptoms related to intestinal dysfunction usually develop when inocula are large. About 10% of patients experience diarrhea within a few days after invasion. This is caused by proliferation of the organisms in the lumen of the intestine prior to and at the time of mucosal penetration [13,23,24,63]. At this stage, the typhoid and paratyphoid fevers resemble the acute gastroenteritis caused by nontyphoidal serotypes. Although free of symptoms, most individuals have transiently positive cultures of the stool early in the course of infections. The organism then disappears from the feces until the active stage of disease has been established (Fig. 8). Fever first appears about one week after exposure, and increases slowly, in stepwise fashion, over several days. This is soon followed by other symptoms, among which are headache (34%), malaise (90%), anorexia (80%), cough (40%), sore throat (20–40%) and muscular-skeletal discomfort (up to 59%) [13,23,63]. Most individuals are characteristically unable to "pinpoint" the exact time at which they first became ill. The disease is often confused with influenza at this stage. From a pathophysiologic standpoint, the clinical manifestations develop at a time in the natural history of the infection when the organisms have penetrated the intestinal mucosa and are multiplying in the lymphoid tissue of the bowel and mesentery and are beginning to gain access to the circulation (Fig. 8).

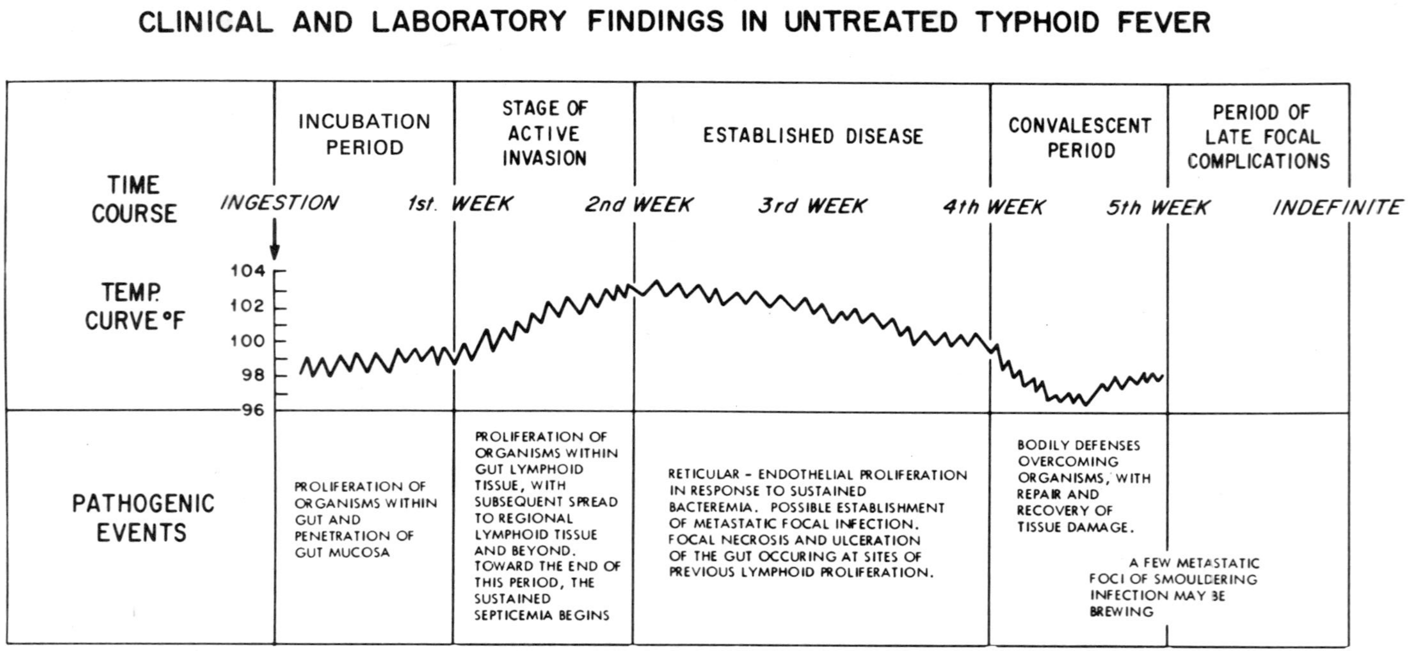

FIG. 8. Time course of clinical, microbiologic, and pathogenic events in untreated typhoid fever. (Continued, facing page.)

DISEASE MANIFESTATIONS	DIARRHEA IN 10–20% OF PATIENTS	HEADACHE MALAISE MYALGIA ANOREXIA NAUSEA COUGH SORE THROAT CONSTIPATION POSSIBLE DIARRHEA	" TOXEMIA " ABDOMINAL DISCOMFORT NEUROPSYCHIATRIC SYNDROMES INTESTINAL ULCERATION GENITO-URINARY SYNDROMES BRONCHITIS RELATIVE BRADYCARDIA SPLENOMEGALY HEPATOMEGALY ROSE SPOTS ANEMIA LEUKOPENIA INTESTINAL PERFORATION AND HEMORRHAGE MAY OCCUR INTERCURRENT RELAPSE MAY OCCUR	DISEASE RELAPSE MAY OCCUR	CHOLECYSTITIS OSTEOMYELITIS SOFT TISSUE ABSCESSES
BLOOD CULTURES	NEGATIVE		80 - 90%	NEGATIVE UNLESS CONTINUED DISEASE OR RELAPSE OCCURS	
STOOL CULTURES	TRANSIENTLY POSITIVE	NEGATIVE	80% POSITIVE	50% POSITIVE	DECREASING INCIDENCE OF POSITIVE CULTURES WITH TIME, 20% AT 2 MONTHS 10% AT 3 MONTHS 3% AT 1 YEAR
URINE CULTURES	NEGATIVE	NEGATIVE	25% POSITIVE	10% POSITIVE	DECREASING INCIDENCE OF POSITIVE CULTURES
ANCILLARY CULTURES { Bone Marrow Rose Spot	NEGATIVE	NEGATIVE	80 - 90% POSITIVE 60% POSITIVE	DECREASING INCIDENCE OF POSITIVE CULTURES	
WIDAL TEST	NEGATIVE	20% POSITIVE	50% POSITIVE	80% POSITIVE	

A number of modes of onset less common than an influenza-like syndrome have been described [144]. Among these is the insidious development of manifestations of neurologic dysfunction, including severe and intractable headache, facial neuralgia, confusion, stupor, maniacal behavior and signs of meningeal irritation—symptoms and signs suggestive of involvement of the central nervous system. Symptoms of dysfunction of the respiratory tract—mild bronchitis, pleurisy or pneumonia—may predominate. Severe vomiting or pain in the right lower quadrant of the abdomen mimicking appendicitis or intestinal hemorrhage or perforation may be the presenting complaints. Rarely, patients may exhibit abnormalities consistent with acute pyelo- or glomerulonephritis; the former is more common.

By the end of the first week of symptoms (two weeks after the ingestion of the organisms), the active phase of the disease is established. At this time, the important clinical manifestations are sustained fever, mental confusion, respiratory and gastrointestinal disburbances, an allegedly characteristic musty, feculent body odor and rose spots on the skin. The incidence of involvement of the respiratory and gastrointestinal tracts in 360 cases of typhoid fever studied at Charity Hospital in New Orleans is presented in Tables 6 and 7. These data underscore the frequency of bronchitis without pneumonia, and the fact that constipation is more common than diarrhea [13]. It has been pointed out that tenderness in the lower abdomen and dilatation of loops of bowel by air and fluid are characteristic findings in this stage of the infection [23,63]. Other physical findings of note include bradycardia relative to the degree of fever during the first week of established disease, splenomegaly (40–60%) and hepatomegaly (approximately 25%) [13,63]. Blood cultures are positive in over 90% of individuals during this period; this reflects the intrusion into the circulation of organisms that have been multiplying in lymphoid tissue. Chills are quite uncommon in uncomplicated enteric fever; their presence suggests a different diagnosis or the development of a complication (Fig. 8) [23,63]. (See Illustrative Case 6, p. 74.)

TABLE 6. Respiratory Manifestations in 360 Cases of Typhoid Fever (modified from Stuart and Pullen [13])

Manifestation	% of cases
Coryza	88
Cough	86
Sore throat	84
Rales	64
Chest pain	60
Cyanosis	36
Epistaxis	21
Pneumonia	11
Pleurisy	2
Pleural effusion	1

TABLE 7. Gastrointestinal Manifestations in 360 Cases of Typhoid Fever (modified from Stuart and Pullen [13])

Manifestation	% of cases
Anorexia	91
Abdominal tenderness	84
Constipation	79
Abdominal distension	76
Foul breath and sordes	69
Nausea and vomiting	54
Diarrhea	43
Gross intestinal hemorrhage	21
Cholecystitis	3
Intestinal perforation	2
Herpes labialis	2
Parotitis	1

An unusual form of typhoid fever is characterized by asymptomatic bacteremia. Patients with this syndrome manifest no symptoms of the disease, but have positive blood cultures. Administration of endotoxins to these individuals produces constitutional signs and symptoms typical of those that usually follow intravenous infusion of the lipopolysaccharide of gram-negative bacteria [273–275]. This syndrome is transient and detected only when culture of the blood is carried out. *Chronic asymptomatic salmonella bacteremia* has been demonstrated in persons with schistosomiasis; they are, however, tolerant to endotoxin [276].

"Rose spots" are slightly raised, discrete, irregular pink macules that blanch on pressure and are 2–4 mm in diameter. They are characteristically present on the anterior aspect of the trunk between the nipples and umbilicus and produce no symptoms. The lesions are occasionally present on the back and arms and rarely on the legs. Rose spots usually appear between the seventh and tenth day of illness. They recur in crops over the next few weeks. Each crop consists of approximately 6–12 macules that gradually involute over 3–4 days and leave no scars. Brawny desquamation of the skin may follow, especially in children [277]. The etiology of these lesions is not clear. It is usually difficult to detect organisms. However, incubation of biopsied tissue in broth for 12–24 hours has yielded *S. typhi,* even in the absence of bacteremia [277–279]. Of 38 patients with typhoid fever and rose spots, many of whom had received antimicrobial agents, the organism could be demonstrated in the lesions of 63% [279]. There is a significant clinical and histologic similarlity between rose spots and the eruption produced by the injection of purified *S. typhi* endotoxin [23]. Although rose spots are said to be present in approximately 30–50% of cases of enteric fever [13,63], they are not specific for this disease. They may also develop in patients with psittacosis [23], leptospirosis [280], brucellosis

[281], rat-bite fever [282], and shigellosis [283]. They are less common in pigmented persons than in Caucasians [13,63,284]. Two recent studies [284,285] of endemic typhoid have indicated that treatment with anti-infective drugs has resulted in a decrease in the incidence of rose spots.

A variety of other lesions of the skin may appear during the acute phase of typhoid fever [144]. A diffuse erythematous flush, *erythema typhosum,* may be present during the first week of the disease. *Erythema nodosum* and *urticaria,* probably manifestations of hypersensitivity, have been described. *Noma* or *dermal gangrene* may develop in the course of typhoid fever, especially in malnourished children. *Transient alopecia areata* is common. *Transverse ridging of the nails* is practically always present. *Herpes labialis* is quite rare, despite the high grade fever that characterizes the enteric fevers.

The clinical course of typhoid fever as well as the useful diagnostic studies, in relation to time, are summarized in Figure 8. Although serologic tests [9–12,16–18] may yield a clue to the possibility of the disease in patients with the syndrome of "fever of unknown origin," isolation of the organism is the *sine qua non* for diagnosis. Gilman has indicated that *S. typhi* may be recovered from the bone marrow (90% of cases) and rose spots (63%) [279]. Cultures of blood, stool and urine were positive in 40, 37 and 7% of patients, respectively. He pointed out that, if only these had been examined, microbiologic proof of typhoid fever would have been available in only 60% of the cases. This experience emphasizes the importance of culture of both bone marrow and lesions in the skin in establishing the diagnosis of the disease, especially if antimicrobial agents have been administered early in its course.

Clinical improvement of untreated typhoid fever characteristically begins between the end of the second week and the fourth week of illness. Defervescence is by gradual lysis rather than crisis (Fig. 8). Various of the "nonfocal" complications, that is, those *not* due to bacteremic dissemination, are most common during this period [13,63]. Among these are gastrointestinal, respiratory, cardiovascular, genito-urinary, hematologic and neuropsychiatric disturbances.

The two most common complications of typhoid fever are intestinal perforation and hemorrhage. Both are related to severe ileal involvement. Each is of prognostic importance. Perforation of the ileum is usually secondary to ulcers situated on the antimesenteric border. Because there is a striking failure of mobilization of the omentum and mesentery, localization of the intestinal contents is poor or absent. This leads to the rapid development of diffuse peritonitis, in many instances. Cultures of peritoneal exudate frequently yield organisms normally present in feces, particularly *E. coli,* rather than *S. typhi.* This may be so because the typhoid bacilli are sequestered within Peyer's patches and other regional lymphoid tissue. Swelling and ulceration of these areas may lead to mucosal necrosis and ulceration, thrombosis of capillaries, and, finally, perforation. This is followed by deposition of the normal microflora of the bowel on the peritoneal surfaces and the development of peritonitis. Ileal hemorrhage may also result from ulceration of lymphoid tissue. Polymorphonuclear leukocytes, in addition to or instead of monocytes, may be present in the wall of a bleeding ulcer, presumably because of the acute necrosis at the site of the lesion [63,286–291].

The incidence of intestinal perforation in the course of typhoid fever is about 2–3% [63,286–290]. The fatality rate in patients who develop this complication is about four times higher than in individuals who do not experience this problem (22% *vs.* 5.4%) [63]. Hemorrhage has been reported to occur in 3% [63] to 21% [13]; the former figure probably reflects life-threatening bleeding because 38% of these cases were fatal. Both intestinal hemorrhage and perforation may present very dramatically and be readily recognizable. However, they may also develop very insidiously in those who are very ill and have abdominal tenderness, anemia and fever. It has been suggested that a sudden increase in the peripheral white blood cell count is an excellent clue to the presence of perforation and peritonitis. Unfortunately, many persons with these complications fail to exhibit this phenomenon [63]. (See Illustrative Cases 7, 8, pp. 75, 76.)

The hepatobiliary system is frequently involved in patients with typhoid fever. Although infection of the bile is the rule in the disease, symptoms suggesting involvement of the gall bladder are usually absent. However, acute cholecystitis may develop in about 2% of cases [13,63]. Acute or chronic cholecystitis may appear months to years after an episode of typhoid fever in some instances; culture of stones and/or bile yields *S. typhi* in such cases. Abscess of the liver due to the typhoid bacillus may develop in patients with obstruction of the biliary tract (292). As pointed out in Chapter III, the histologic features of the livers of patients with this syndrome are "Mallory nodules," hypertrophy and proliferation of the Kupffer cells, focal necrosis of nests of hepatocytes and portal infiltration with lymphocytes. Biochemical studies indicate the presence of cholestasis. The transaminases (SGOT and SGPT) are minimally to moderately increased, levels of circulating bilirubin are elevated (usually less than 7 mg/dcl) and concentrations of alkaline phosphatase in serum range from 1.5 to 3 times the normal value. The pathogenesis of the hepatic dysfunction is not clear. Cholangitis is not present. Possible reasons for these abnormalities are (a) nonspecific reaction to the presence of any type of bacterial infection, (b) a specific effect of *S. typhi* and (c) co-existing viral hepatitis acquired simultaneously with the typhoid bacilli from contaminated food or water. The latter is highly possible because breaks in sanitation and the fecal-oral route of transmission are common critical factors in the spread of both the viral and bacterial diseases. Rarely, typhoid patients have been reported to develop hepatic failure [13,63,293–296].

Anorexia and nausea are universal symptoms of typhoid fever. Constipation is more common than diarrhea; the latter is not related to the degree of anatomical abnormality of the intestine or to the risk of perforation or hemorrhage.

The severity of the untreated disease, the marked degree of debilitation produced by it and the commonly present poor hygiene predispose patients with typhoid to the development of suppurative parotitis. The agent most commonly involved in this complication is *S. aureus*. Gram-negative enteric organisms as well as members of the normal oral microflora may be responsible, in some instances. *S. typhi* is only rarely involved.

Patients with typhoid fever, like those with any disorder associated with protracted fever, may complain bitterly of discomfort in the tongue. Osler has described this vividly [144]:

> Early in the disease it is moist, swollen and coated with a thin white fur, which, as the fever progresses, becomes dense. It may remain moist throughout. It is small in size and tends to be red at the edge and tip. In severe cases, particularly those with delirium, the tongue becomes very dry, partly owing to the fact that such patients breathe with the mouth open. It may be covered with a brown or brownish-black fur or with crusts between which are cracks and fissures. . . . In these cases, the teeth and lips may be covered with a dark brownish matter called *sordes*—a mixture of food, epithelial debris, and micro-organisms. By keeping the mouth and tongue clean from the outset the fissures, which are extremely painful, may be prevented. During convalescence the tongue eventually becomes clearer and the fur thrown off, almost imperceptibly or occasionally "in flakes."

Subtle gastrointestinal disturbances may appear during the course of typhoid fever. Mild impairment of small bowel function is demonstrable even during convalescence. Malabsorption of D-xylose is present in about 50% of patients during this period; this is not the case for fat [297,298]. Because absorption of D-xylose normally takes place in the upper part of the small intestine [299], there is good correlation with the anatomic lesion in the jejunum [134]. Pancreatitis, not related to metastatic infection, may develop rarely [300].

Manifestations of dysfunction of the upper respiratory tract and of bronchitis are the rule in typhoid fever (Table 6). Epistaxis is common. Pleurisy is rare. "Typhoid lobar pneumonia," the etiology of which is not clear, has been noted in 1 to 8% of cases. *S. typhi* has been recovered from the sputum in only a few instances. Pneumonia due to *Streptococcus pneumoniae* is more common. It appears very likely that the debility and possibly the bronchitis caused by the typhoid bacillus in untreated patients leads to an increase in the risk of invasion and infection of the lungs by organisms that colonize the upper airway. This is analogous to the nosocomial pneumonitides known to occur in individuals with other types of severely debilitating illness. Although pneumonia may be present early in the course of typhoid fever, it usually appears insidiously late in the disease [18,63,301]. Other complications involving the respiratory tract are presently quite uncommon. Although edema, ulceration and perforation of the larynx and perichondritis have been reported in the past, they are presently very rare. Paralysis of the muscles of the larynx still occurs. This is presumed to be due to involvement of the laryngeal nerves, and is often associated with evidence of other types of neurologic dysfunction.

"Toxic" myocarditis develops in 1–2% of patients with severe typhoid fever. The clinical features are cardiomegaly, various types of arrhythmia, and congestive failure associated with a low output state. The electrocardiographic abnormalities are those present in other kinds of cardiomyopathy and include prolongation of conduction (increased PR and QT intervals), varying degrees of block, changes in T waves and ST segments, and atrial and ventricular arrhythmias; some or all of these may be present. The pathoanatomic findings include necrosis, degeneration and fatty infiltration of myocardial cells. Whether or not the characteristic relative bradycardia of typhoid fever is a manifestation of clinically inapparent myocarditis is unknown. It must be emphasized that tachycardia is fairly common in the second and third week of the disease. Bacterial invasion is clearly not the cause of the myocardial involvement. The pathogenetic mechanisms responsible for this syndrome have not been defined [12,63,290,302–305]. Other cardiovascular complications include pericarditis [306], peripheral vascular collapse and venous and arterial thrombosis; the latter is thought to be related to the low output, congestive failure and prolonged confinement in bed [13,63].

About 25% of patients excrete *S. typhi* in the urine during the acute stage of the disease [63]; chronic urinary carriage may also occur. At least one case of xanthogranulomatous pyelonephritis complicating typhoid fever has been reported [307]. Prostatitis, epidymitis and/or orchitis may develop, and may recur when the organism is present in the urine. It has recently become apparent that the deposition of immune complexes, consisting of specific antibody, third component of complement and Vi antigen, in the basement membranes of kidney glomeruli may lead to the development of glomerulonephritis. Transient proteinuria has been noted to be the only urinary abnormality in some patients with typhoid fever in whom the presence of this glomerular lesion was demonstrated by renal biopsy [149]. It has been suggested that immune complex-complement-mediated tissue damage may be more common than has been appreciated in other infections in which protein is transiently present in the urine [308]. It probably also explains the cases of severe glomerulonephritis that have been noted occasionally in individuals with enteric fever [282,293,309], and perhaps other poorly understood complications of this disease, such as myocarditis, hepatitis, nonsuppurative arthritis and some of the neuropsychiatric disorders. Interstitial nephritis progressing to renal failure [63] and the hemolytic-uremic syndrome [310] are rare complications of typhoid fever.

Spontaneous abortion and premature labor are common in untreated pregnant patients with typhoid fever [13]. Puerperal sepsis may develop when the disease occurs at the time of labor and delivery. Treatment of this infection during pregnancy with ampicillin (for 14 days), but not chloramphenicol because of the risk of fetal toxicity, has been found to reduce strikingly the incidence of miscarriage [311].

The commonest hematologic abnormality observed in patients with typhoid fever is anemia. This is probably due to blood loss and suppression of the bone marrow by the infection. A significant degree of hemolysis has been noted in individuals with glucose-6-phosphate dehydrogenase deficiency of the erythrocytes [312–320]. Although it has been assumed that this is probably related to treatment with chloramphenicol [312–317], it has been shown that it is primarily due to the infectious process and that the antibiotic exerts only a minor additive or synergistic effect [318–320]. Leukopenia and eosinopenia are common. The peripheral white blood count may be decreased to less than 2,000/mm^3. In the second or third week it may be increased to 12,000/mm^3 or higher; this suggests the possibility of metastatic infection or intestinal perforation [24,63]. Abnormalities of the clotting mechanism have also been noted in typhoid fever. Two instances of disseminated intravascular coagulation [293,321] and of the hemolytic-uremic syndrome [310] have been reported in patients with the disease. Of interest is the regular occurrence of a polyclonal increase in the concentration of serum globulins; this is often associated with the appearance of rheumatoid factor in high titer. These abnormalities, like the others, disappear with effective chemotherapy [322].

Fever, headache, malaise, myalgia, anorexia, nausea, leukopenia, thrombopenia, activation of complement and the coagulation cascade and stimulation of the hypothalamic-pituitary-adrenal axis are phenomena common to the activity of endotoxin (lipopolysaccharide, LPS) and the clinical syndrome of enteric fever. For this reason, it has been suggested that LPS plays an important role in the pathophysiology of typhoid fever. However, this has been questioned by Hornick and his colleagues [26] on the basis of the results of incisive investigations in which fever was used as the indicator of the effect of the lipopolysaccharide. They studied two groups of volunteers, one tolerant and the other nontolerant to endotoxin who were inoculated with living *S. typhi*. The clinical picture developing in both groups was the same. Hypersensitivity to catecholamines, common in typhoid fever, was present in both the tolerant and nontolerant subjects. Although these observations are highly suggestive of lack of a role of LPS in the pathogenesis of enteric fever, this possibility has not been completely eliminated. It is possible that endotoxin may modify or enhance the inflammatory response at sites of multiplication of the organisms in the intestine. The lipopolysaccharide may exert different effects when it is contained within the bacterial cell wall than when it is in the "free state." Antibody to the R-core of endotoxin appears to protect against the activity of LPS and also against the effects of bacteremia due to some gram-negative bacilli [27]. Similar studies of the lipopolysaccharide of the typhoid bacillus may provide a better understanding of its role in enteric fever and possibly offer a new approach to the therapy of this disease.

It has become apparent in recent years that neuropsychiatric disturbances may be a prominent feature of typhoid fever, particularly in individuals living in developing countries [323–326]. Confusional states as well as acute schizophrenia have been described with great regularity among African patients, especially those without much formal education [323,324,327]. Although toxic encephalopathy is common in typhoid fever occurring in any area of the world, acute psychotic episodes, even in the absence of elevated temperature initially, is a frequent presenting symptom among this cultural group. The manifestations clear with antimicrobial therapy [323,324]. Among other neurologic complications unrelated to focal metastatic infection are encephalomyelitis (histologic features identical to those in post-viral encephalitis) (325), transverse myelitis [326], Guillain-Barré syndrome [328] and cranial and peripheral neuropathy [323–326]. Whether these are causally related to the basic infection or to unidentified intercurrent processes is not clear. It has become evident, nevertheless, that neuropsychiatric manifestations are presently much more common than they appear to have been in the past. Gulati and his colleagues [284] have recently pointed out that intestinal hemorrhage and perforation have been replaced by peripheral vascular collapse and encephalopathic disorders as the most frequent complications of typhoid fever.

Severe otitis media associated with transient decrease in auditory acuity may complicate typhoid fever. Among the ocular manifestations that have been observed in the course of this infection are conjunctivitis (often accompanied by keratitis and uveitis), dysfunction of the extraocular muscles, thrombosis of the orbital veins, and cataracts (usually follows involvement of the uveal tract). Some of these may leave permanent residua [144].

Relapse is a well-known complication of typhoid fever. It occurs in both treated (with antibiotic agents) and untreated patients; the incidence in the latter ranges from 3 to 13%. There is some evidence that the incidence of this phenomenon is not reduced by the utilization of effective antimicrobial drugs; it even has been suggested that the relapse rate is increased by such therapy. Two types of relapse have been recognized; (a) one that develops after convalescence has been established, and (b) another "intermittent relapse," that occurs while symptoms and signs of the disease are still present but are decreased in intensity. That multiple relapses may occur is illustrated by a case described by Osler [144], in which the illness extended over a period of 11 months and was characterized by six episodes of recurrence of active infection. The relapsing disease may be more severe, in all aspects, than the initial syndrome, and be complicated by intestinal hemorrhage or perforation, metastatic infection and other manifestations.

Because sustained bacteremia is a universal feature of typhoid fever, metastatic infections due to the *S. typhi* may appear during the acute or convalescent stage of the disease, or months to years after full recovery. Any area of the body may be involved. The commonest sites are bones (extremities, spine and ribs). Focalization may also occur in the spleen, muscles, breasts, thyroid, cervical lymph nodes, salivary glands and abdominal cavity. A more detailed discussion of focal infections complicating salmonellosis, in general, is presented below.

The clinical syndromes of the enteric fevers in patients under 5 years of age are frequently different from those in older youngsters and adults. A wider range of serotypes of salmonella is involved in the young children. Nonspecific manifestations of infections, including fever, convulsions, diarrhea or vomiting, are common major presenting complaints. The child who lives in a tropical area may remain afebrile despite the presence of bacteremia; high grade fever and rigors may develop following blood transfusion [258,329].

It is impossible, in individual instances, to determine whether a given episode of enteric fever is due to *S. typhi* or to another species of salmonella. However, study of large numbers of cases has indicated that the vast majority are caused by typhoid and paratyphoid bacilli. A study of 2,647 untreated cases has documented the fact that typhoid fever is the most severe form of the disease [272]. The mean duration of fever, fatality rare, incidence of relapse, intestinal hemorrhage and perforation of the bowel with peritonitis were noted to be 30.2 days, 18.5%, 12.5% and 14.1%, respectively, when *S. typhi* was involved. When paratyphoid bacilli were responsible for the infection, these figures were 20.7 days, 3.5%, 4.4% and 9%, respectively.

SALMONELLA BACTEREMIA (SEPTICEMIA)

Organisms may be present transiently in the blood of patients with gastroenteritis caused by salmonella. They persist for longer periods in the circulation of individuals with one of the forms of enteric fever. The following features of bacteremia associated with invasion by nontyphoidal salmonella have been defined by Cherubin et al. [191]. It has a bimodal age distribution, and is most common in children who experience transient and insignificant intrusion of organisms into the circulation in the course of acute gastroenteritis. It has been suggested that *S. heidelberg* and *S. virchow* may be especially invasive in this age group, especially neonates [105,258,330]. Temporary invasion of the bloodstream also occurs in adults with primary infection of the intestine. High grade sustained bacteremia may be a problem in the presence of such underlying disorders as lymphoproliferative disease, sickle cell anemia, etc. The fatality rate in these individuals with nontyphoidal bacteremia is about 13.3%. However, in few cases is salmonellosis the established cause of death. The major significance of the presence of salmonella in the blood in persons with no other illness is the predisposition to the establishment of metastatic focal infections. This is more important than the direct septic consequences of the transient appearance of the organism in the circulation.

Chronic bacteremia is the primary feature of the syndrome of *salmonella bacteremia* (*septicemia*). The responsible bacteria establish themselves in the intestinal tract only uncommonly. A number of other features distinguish this type of disease from other kinds of salmonellosis. Among these are (a) causative serotypes limited in number and different from those that produce acute enteritis or typhoid-paratyphoid fever, (b) a higher incidence (8 to 10%) of metastatic infection, (c) a preponderance in men over 50 years of age, and (d) association with special predisposing factors, including acute hemolytic processes, atherosclerotic aneurysms of the aorta and its main branches, valvular heart disease, the presence of neoplastic disease and others.

S. choleraesuis is the prototype of the salmonella that causes *salmonella bacteremia* [331]. This species was, until recently, the species most frequently responsible for this syndrome, despite the fact that it is not among the 10 serotypes involved most often in the pathogenesis of salmonellosis (Table 3) [332,333]. Because of strict control of the production and distribution of pork products in the United States over the past few years, this is no longer the case. However, this organism is still the most prone to invade the bloodstream, even when it causes other clinical forms of salmonellosis [191]. The fatality rate of infections produced by *S. choleraesuis* are 2 to 3 times higher than that of typhoid fever, and at least 5 to 6 times greater than that of disease caused by other serotypes. Metastatic infectious foci, the most important of which are intravascular lesions, osteomyelitis and meningitis, are common complications of disease due to this serotype [271,332–334]. The organism may lie dormant in some tissues, usually bone, for many years and then become active and produce infection [251,333]. An extreme example of this phenomenon is the report of a blood donor with longstanding asymptomatic bacteremia with *S. choleraesuis,* transfusion of whose blood to a number of healthy individuals resulted in an extended outbreak of disease due to this organism in the recipients [111]. Allison and his colleagues [333] have pointed out that the pathogenesis of salmonellosis due to *S. choleraesuis* is still vague. "The high virulence of this organism, the low level of intestinal pathogenicity is most puzzling. That even gastrointestinal subclinical infection is probably rare is borne out by the low level of carriers. Yet, paradoxically, this organism has been demonstrated to survive for years outside of the patient's gastrointestinal tract and to produce repeated bouts of clinical disease." *S. typhimurium* is the serotype presently responsible most often for salmonella bacteremia. This is, in part, related to the fact that it is the most frequent cause of infection in animals and man and, in part, to its relatively high invasive capacity. *S. enteritidis, S. heidelberg* and *S. oranienberg* have been increasingly involved in the pathogenesis of this syndrome in recent years [105].

Documentation of high grade bacteremia, as indicated by more than 50% of blood cultures being persistently positive for the putative organisms in the course of nontyphoidal salmonellosis, strongly suggests the presence of intravascular focal infection. This is especially characteristic of infections caused by *S. choleraesuis* and *S. typhimurium.* Two major foci are involved, the endothelium of large arteries and the endocardium. The former may result in the development of a true or pseudo-aneurysm, usually of the abdominal or descending thoracic aorta or the iliofemoral vessels [251,335–353]. However, it must be emphasized that, in a great majority of instances of the syndrome of *salmonella bacteremia,* an atherosclerotic aneurysm is present for months or years prior to infection by salmonella. This lesion may be infected by the organisms, especially if a sterile clot is present. Interestingly, one of us (L.W.) has observed a small number of cases in which no evidence of inflammatory reaction was detected in the aneurysmal wall. Involvement of the endocardium leads to endocarditis with extensive valvular damage, thrombosis, development of myocardial abscesses that may perforate the ventricle and aneurysms of the sinus of Valsalva or ventricular wall.

The large elastic arteries are normally quite resistant to infection [337–339]. However, as is the case with valvular lesions, the presence of acquired or congenital abnormalities of the vessels increases their susceptibility to bacterial invasion to a high degree [251,339,340]. Vascular sites other than aneurysms of arteries on which salmonella may be implanted are patent ductus arteriosus, coarctation of the aorta [354], arteriovenous fistula [355], coronary arteritis [356], idiopathic cystic medial necrosis [357], syphilitic arteritis [336], a Hufnagel valve [358] and normal thoracic aorta [359]. Of 21 patients with *salmonella bacteremia,* in which invasion of an abdominal aortic aneurysm had occurred, 17 were noted to have atherosclerotic changes in the vessel [335], 19 died. The major cause of death was rupture of the undisturbed infected aneurysm, or a tear at the suture line in individuals in whom a graft had been placed. Seven of the cases were due to *S. choleraesuis* and 2 to members of group C, possibly *S. choleraesuis*; 6 were caused by *S. typhimurium* and the other 6 by other serotypes. In contrast to the gravity of the disease of the aorta induced by these organisms, invasion of more distal vessels, particularly the femoral and popliteal arteries, has been associated with an excellent prognosis; 7 of 8 patients with this type of involvement have been reported to have survived following surgical excision of the lesion [349,350]. *Staphylococcus aureus* and *salmonella species* (primarily *S. choleraesuis* and *S. typhimurium*) are the most common causes of bacterial infections of major arteries [350,353].

Several potential mechanisms are involved in the pathogenesis of invasion of arterial aneurysms by salmonella [251,341,348,352,353,360]: (a) *Primary* or *cryptogenic mycotic aneurysm*; in these, a suppurative arteritis develops in the absence of an infection at other sites in the cardiovascular system. The aneurysm is usually situated at a site of atherosclerotic degeneration and becomes infected in the course of an episode of transient intrusion of *S. choleraesuis* or *S. typhimurium* into the bloodstream. (b) *Secondary or embolomycotic aneurysm*; suppuration in the arterial wall is the result of embolic spread of organisms from another infected area such as other vessels or the heart, most often endocarditis, to the intima or the vasa vasorum. (c) *Mycotic aneurysm secondary to direct extension*; infection of surrounding soft tissues of bone spreads contiguously or via lymphatics to the arterial wall. A particularly interesting example of this type of disease is the association of salmonella osteomyelitis of the lumbar spine with accompanying paravertebral abscess and a secondarily infected atherosclerotic aortic aneurysm [250,251,342,361]. It has been postulated that pressure exerted by the uninfected dilated area of the aorta on an adjacent vertebral body produces necrosis of bone that then serves as a site for invasion by the organisms; the development of a paravertebral abscess is followed by direct spread of the bacteria to the aneurysm [250,251]. (d) *Established atherosclerotic aneurysm that is unrelated to invasion by salmonella.* The lesion may or may not contain a sterile thrombus that may have been present for some time before infection occurs. If a clot is present, this is invaded in the course of the bacteremia; if it is absent, the organism may penetrate the aneurysmal walls. In some instances, there is no evidence of infection of the aneurysm.

The interval between onset of invasion by salmonella and erosion and rupture of an involved artery is unpredictable. Three syndromes may develop in the course of this type of infection. (a) A diffuse suppurative arteritis may develop and be followed by rupture and the appearance of a saccular or false aneurysm. (b) The arteritis may be focal and lead to the same consequences as the diffuse type. (c) Secondary infection may occur and result in expansion, erosion and perforation of a preexisting aneurysm [348,352,353]. Debilitated elderly patients, individuals with the highest frequency of atherosclerosis and the greatest risk of the development of aneurysms, have been noted to be especially susceptible to *salmonella bacteremia.* The risk of this is increased by surgical manipulation and the presence of neoplastic disorders or debilitating systemic disorders [363,364].

The presence of certain clinical features suggest the possibility of arterial infections due to salmonella. Among these are (a) persistent fever following gastroenteritis in patients with a palpable aneurysm, (b) pain in the back, abdomen, or chest in the face of bacteremia with salmonella, (c) reappearance of the bacteria in the blood during or after a prolonged course of effective therapy, (d) intrusion of the organisms into the circulation of individuals with a vascular graft or prosthesis, (e) vertebral osteomyelitis associated with bacteremia, especially if a paravertebral mass is present, (f) an unexplained large number of salmonella in the bloodstream, and (g) prolonged fever after a documented episode of gastroenteritis [349,350]. (See Illustrative Cases 10, 11, pp 78, 81.)

The incidence of cardiac infections due to salmonella is lower than that of arterial aneurysms [365,366]. Certain features characterize involvement of the heart by this group of organisms. The serotypes most often involved are *S. choleraesuis* and *S. typhimurium*. Previously diseased mitral and aortic valves are the commonest sites of implantation of the bacteria. Calcified ventricular aneurysms or pre-existing mural thrombi may also be colonized in some cases; this is unusual. Endocarditis caused by salmonella is frequently acute, and may be complicated by atrial thrombosis, extensive valvular perforation and destruction, pericarditis, pancarditis and myocardial abscess. Fatality rates are high, even after appropriate antimicrobial therapy [365–376]. Endocardial infection and mycotic aneurysms may be present simultaneously [341,377].

It has been suggested that cardiac surgery, anesthesia, hypotension, stress ulcers of the intestinal tract and prophylactic use of antibiotics may lead to conversion of asymptomatic carriage of salmonella in the bowel to active clinical disease with bacteremia and focalization of the organism [378]. A case has been reported in which transient intrusion of *S. typhimurium* into the blood led to invasion along a transvenous cardiac pacemaker and infective mural endocarditis [379].

McNally et al. [370] have suggested that infection of the heart by salmonella differs significantly from other forms of endocarditis in a number of aspects. There is a relatively high incidence of *mural endocarditis,* and atypical sites such as the lining of ventricular aneurysms, the area of ventricle overlying a syphilitic process, the wall of a sclerotic (rheumatic) atrium, and atrial mural thrombi are frequently involved. Although infective endocarditis caused by salmonella may respond favorably to treatment with antibiotics, this is not the case in most patients [368,380]. McNally and his colleagues (370) have suggested that endocarditis due to these organisms closely resembles the endarteritis commonly produced by them, and that the reason for this is the unusual propensity of salmonella to attack mural surfaces in the heart and arteries. The implications of this concept for therapy are clear. Because antimicrobial therapy alone is inadequate for the management of arterial infection [335–353,370], it probably also fails to alter the course of cardiac involvement. It is likely that chemotherapy together with surgery holds the greatest promise of cure. This has recently been emphasized by a report of recovery of a case of endocarditis due to salmonella by the administration of antibiotics and replacement of the infected valve by a prosthesis [381]. (See Illustrative Case 12, p. 83.)

FOCAL INFECTIONS CAUSED BY SALMONELLA

The first instance of osteomyelitis complicating typhoid fever was recorded by Paget in 1876 [328]. Since then, it has been established that involvement of bone develops in approximately 0.8% of patients with disease due to *S. typhi* [383]; in 0.2% of those infected by *S. schottmulleri* [384] and in a smaller number of those in whom other serotypes are involved. Osteomyelitis that occurs in instances of salmonellosis other than enteric fever is most often caused by *S. choleraesuis* and *S. typhimurium* [385]. This reflects the high incidence of bacteremia associated with invasion by these serotypes. Sickle cell anemia increases the risk of infection of bone by salmonella [386]. Salmonella infection accounts for less than 1.0% of the cases of hematogenous osteomyelitis occurring in otherwise healthy individuals [387–390].

Any area of the skeleton may be invaded by salmonella. However, the long bones (especially the proximal humerus and distal femur), chondrosternal junctions and spine are most frequently infected [251,391]. Although the metaphysis is commonly affected when osteomyelitis is caused by other organisms, invasion by salmonella usually involves the diaphysis and epiphysis. There is a high incidence of pyarthrosis [251,384,392]. More than one vertebra is usually invaded simultaneously when the vertebral space is attacked. The process may be located in either the neural arch and its appendages or, more frequently, in the vertebral body; mediastinal or paravertebral abscess is a frequent complication of this kind of disease [251]. Spondylitis due to this group of organisms is largely self-limited, and is associated with a tendency to spontaneous fusion of the affected vertebrae [393,394]. The radiographic appearance of the affected sites in the spine may resemble that produced by tuberculosis; the disc spaces are involved early and osseous lesions appear later [251]. Multiple bones are infected in about 15% of cases of osteomyelitis caused by salmonella; this is much more common than when the process is produced by other bacteria [251,384]. Salmonella may be introduced directly into bone at sites of trauma [395], or invade areas in which fractures, prostheses, metal plates or screws are present [396,397]. (See Illustrative Cases 9, 16, pp. 77, 87.)

Two types of arthritis may develop in patients with salmonellosis: (a) Bacteremia may result in focalization in a joint; the process is suppurative, and organisms are usually present in the fluid (392). (b) A sterile inflammatory reaction may involve the synovia; this usually occurs as a complication of gastroenteritis caused by salmonella [398–400]. Suppurative arthritis develops in about 0.2–0.3% of all forms of salmonellosis [250,401]. Its incidence is 2.4% when infection is caused by *S. choleraesuis*. Ten per cent of all cases of this complication of salmonellosis are due to this serotype [332]. About 55% of the patients are less than 6 years old; most are younger than 12 months of age. The knees, shoulders, hips and sacroiliac joints are most commonly affected [392]. Two mechanisms are involved in the pathogenesis of invasion of joint spaces by salmonella. These are (a) direct inoculation by organisms circulating in the blood, and (b) primary infection of bone, especially the epiphysis in young children, followed by contiguous spread to the synovia [251,392]. The frequency of bacteremia associated with disease caused by *S. choleraesuis* and *S. typhimurium* explains the high frequency with which these are responsible for complications involving the skeletal system.

Nonsuppurative arthritis is more common than the suppurative form in disease due to salmonella. It occurs in about 2.5% of cases of gastroenteritis due to this group of organisms. Transient diarrhea usually precedes involvement of the joints by some weeks. The clinical presentation may mimic Reiter's syndrome, in some instances; however, urethritis is usually absent [398–400]. *S. typhimurium* is the serotype most frequently involved.

The first case of meningitis caused by salmonella was reported by Ghon in 1907 [402]. The incidence of this complication of salmonellosis appears to be lower than the 1% reported by Saphra and Winter [250]. This type of meningeal disease is six times more common in children than in adults; ¾ of the patients are under 2 years of age; most cases occur in the neonatal period [78,250,251,403–405]. Three large epidemics of meningitis due to this group of bacteria have occurred in newborn nurseries [406–408]. The organisms most often responsible for meningeal infection in youngsters less than 6 years of age are *E. coli*, group B streptococci and salmonella. The reasons for the predisposition of neonates to meningitis caused by these species are not entirely clear; premature birth and the accompanying immaturity of immunologic mechanisms, increased permeability of the blood-brain barrier, and obstetrical trauma have been thought to play a role [409–412]. The serotypes of salmonella most often involved are *S. choleraesuis, S. typhimurium, S. enteritidis* and *S. schottmulleri* [404,413]. Although *S. panama* and *S. habana* account for a considerable number of the cases recorded in the world's literature, they have, for the most part, been implicated in a few epidemics in nurseries [407,408]. There is no evidence that infection by these types of salmonella increases the risk of spread to the meninges. The clinical and pathoanatomic features of meningitis produced by salmonella do not differ from those present in other pyogenic meningitides [251,405]. However, basilar accumulation of the inflammatory exudate and hydrocephalus are more frequent with the former [404,414]. (See Illustrative Case 5, p. 73.)

As is the case with *S. aureus*, the circulation of salmonella in the blood is associated with metastatic infection of a large number of extravascular sites, and leads to the development of both microscopic and macroscopic abscesses. The serotypes that invade the bloodstream and produce focal infections most often are *S. typhi, S. choleraesuis, S. typhimurium* and *S. schottmulleri*. Among the localized lesions that have been observed are abscess of the breast (0.3–0.5% of all typhoid patients, and approximately 0.9% of women with typhoid [415]), neonatal suppurative mastitis [416,417], skin [63,418], and testes [419,420]. Salmonella, when they circulate in the blood, may also focalize in subdural hematomas [421,422], ascitic fluid [423], inflammed pancreas [424], cysts [425], tumors [251,426–429] and amebic abscesses [430]. Other metastatic foci include abscesses of the lung [431], spleen [432], subphrenic space [433], adrenal [434], pleural sac [435,436] and other areas [144,251]. An interesting instance of infection of a leg by *S. typhimurium* in which "gas" was present has been described by David and his colleagues [437]. Localization of infection is most likely to develop in tissues that are abnormal or devitalized; this accounts, in some instances, for their unusual locations. (See Illustrative Cases 13, 14, 15, pp. 85, 86.)

THE SALMONELLA CARRIER STATE

Development of the asymptomatic carrier state in the course of infections caused by salmonella results from the interplay of several factors. Among these are the number of organisms involved in initiating the disease, the characteristics of the etiologic serotype, the presence of disorders of the renal and biliary systems and the functional state of the defense mechanisms of the patient. Although carriage of salmonella is most often a consequence of active disease due to these organisms, it may also appear in individuals who, although infected, are not ill [62]. Exposure to inocula of the bacteria too small to produce disease is particularly conducive to induction of the carrier state [114]. Although acute gastroenteritis is said to be the most commonly *recognized* syndrome caused by salmonella, data obtained from a few well studied outbreaks of nontyphoidal salmonellosis suggest that the transient asymptomatic carrier states may be even more common [438,439]. An unusually detailed investigation of a large epidemic (745 cases) of disease due to *S. newport* in Sweden in 1960 indicated that 65.8% of the patients exhibited only carriage of the organism; about 2% developed severe life-threatening illness, and the others had typical gastroenteritis. Individuals with possible exposure, even if asymptomatic, were actively sought out and studied microbiologically. It is very likely that similar observations will be made in outbreaks that are subjected to the same degree of highly precise and detailed clinical and bacteriologic monitoring as was carried out in the Swedish study [438,439].

All patients with gastroenteritis due to salmonella excrete the organisms early in the course of the disease; as many as 10^6 to 10^9/gm are present in the feces. The bacteria can be recovered from stools in 92.5% of cases after 2 weeks, in 41% after 4, in 17.2% after 9, in 11.6% after 10 and in 4.7% after 20 weeks. Individuals are considered "chronic salmonella carriers" if they continue to excrete bacilli one year or more after infection. This is the situation in about 0.2–0.6% of persons with disease due to nontyphoidal serotypes. Whether the initial active disease has been asymptomatic or symptomatic plays no role in determining the duration of persistence of salmonella in the intestine [60,61,250,440].

The organisms responsible for typhoid and paratyphoid fever are recoverable from stool in the vast majority of patients 7 to 10 days after the disease begins, but usually not earlier than this. They are present in the feces of 50% of cases after one month, in 20% after two and in 10% after three months. The incidence of chronic carriage (one year or longer) of *S. typhi* and *S. paratyphi* is about 3% [63,441–444]. Whether chronic carriage of typhoidal and nontyphoidal salmonella is constant or intermittent is still a matter of controversy [25,26,73,441–448]. There is also no agreement on valid criteria for determining the end of the carrier state. Three negative cultures of stool have been accepted, in general, as defining the end point by most physicians; others require that the cultures be free of the organisms for one year.

A number of factors involved in the pathogenesis of chronic carriage of salmonella have been identified. Age plays an important role. Children less than one year old tend to be prolonged convalescent carriers; they usually do not develop the chronic state [60,61]. Individuals in the sixth decade of life have the highest rate of carriage; about 10% of those who have had typhoid fever (especially women) excrete the organisms for prolonged periods [62]. It has been pointed out that this age and sex distribution for the chronic carrier state parallels that of cholelithiasis [443,449]. The administration of pancreozymin to chronic carriers of *S. typhi* regularly produces release of viable organisms into the duodenum, presumably via the common bile duct [450]. The biliary tree is thought to be the site of multiplication of salmonella, especially the serotypes that cause enteric fever, in patients who continue to excrete the bacilli. Difficulty in eradication of the carrier state is related to the presence of stones and chronic inflammation in this area [449–451]. Recurrent episodes of acute cholangitis have been observed in a patient with Caroli's syndrome (multiple intrahepatic biliary cysts) who harbored *S. heidelberg* in the biliary tract [452]. The number of salmonella in carriers is usually large (10^6–10^9/gm of feces). Symptoms are usually not present; the reason for this is not clear.

Chronic carriage of salmonella in the urinary tract is related to the presence of obstructive uropathy due to stones, strictures, tumor or hydronephrosis, to tuberculosis or schistosomiasis. Attempts to eradicate the organisms by treatment with antimicrobial agents are usually futile until the underlying anatomic problems are corrected [276,428,453–455].

SALMONELLA INFECTIONS COMPLICATING OTHER ILLNESSES

Salmonellosis may develop in the course of other types of severe illness [250,251]. One study of a group of 95 cases of infection caused by this group of organisms has revealed that 74% of adults and 27% of children had another unrelated disorder [456]. Other reports have indicated an incidence of 40% of underlying disease that may have predisposed to invasion by salmonella [457,458]. About 46% of the bacteremias caused by these bacilli have occurred in patients with other systemic illness [459]. Although atherosclerosis and malnutrition appear to increase susceptibility, the most common predisposing factors are *"blockade" of the reticuloendothelial system (RES), neoplastic disease, schistosomiasis and inflammatory bowel disease.*

Blockade of the RES. In a comprehensive review of unusual aspects of salmonellosis, Black and his colleagues have pointed out at least four disorders featured by blockade of reticuloendothelial cells that predispose to this infection. These are sicle cell anemia, malaria, bartonellosis and louse-borne relapsing fever [251]. Hemolysis, characteristic of the first three, imposes a heavy burden upon the RES. The organisms themselves may block and depress phagocytic function in louse-borne relapsing fever.

Hodges and Holt were the first to report that sickle cell anemia and other hemoglobinopathies predispose to infection of bones by salmonella [273]. This observation has been confirmed by others [79,251,385,460–467]. Osteomyelitis due to this group of organisms is commonest in young children, especially boys with SS hemoglobinopathy. The serotype most often involved is *S. typhimurium.* The disease usually affects multiple long bones, but may be restricted to the vertebral column (with or without accompanying paravertebral abscess) or to the hands and feet; the latter is most frequent in infants, while the other two forms occur primarily in older children. Although individuals with sickle cell anemia produce adequate concentrations of specific antibody following exposure to antigens of salmonella [468], and there is no evidence that bacterial multiplication in the blood is excessive [463], their ability to resist infection is, nevertheless, decreased. Hook and his colleagues have suggested that blockade of the RES as a result of phagocytosis by macrophages of the breakdown products of the hemolytic process reduces the capacity of these cells to ingest and kill salmonella [469–474]. It is not surprising, therefore, that bacteremia in patients with sickle cell disease is very often caused by these organisms [78]. This may be related to thrombosis of intestinal blood vessels induced by the sickling process, which then leads to easy access of salmonella to the systemic circulation. Thrombotic aseptic infarction of bone is probably the mechanism responsible for the high frequency of osteomyelitis due to this group of organisms in persons with this hemoglobinopathy [251]; sickle crises often precede the invasion of the bone by the salmonellae [78]. (See Illustrative Case 18, p. 89.)

The processes involved in predisposing patients with sickle cell anemia to salmonellosis also serve to increase susceptibility to this infection in those with malaria, relapsing fever and bartonellosis [78,251]. Invasion by salmonella may complicate the therapy of neurosyphilis with malaria [78] and may become common during epidemics of the plasmodial disease [78,475]. Similar relations exist with relapsing fever [475,476] and bartonellosis [477–479]; 40% of cases of the latter develop salmonellosis, most frequently during the hemolytic phase, and the fatality rate is high.

Neoplastic Disease. A number of factors are known to alter the susceptibility of patients with neoplastic disease to invasion by salmonella. Among these are (a) an increase in the possibility of exposure to the organisms, (b) impaired local resistance, (c) abnormalities in phagocytic function and cellular and/or humoral immunity, and (d) immunosuppression by the drugs used to treat the malignant disease [427,429,459,480]. There is a greater risk of exposure to these organisms in individuals with cancers and other neoplasms because of their need for frequent and often prolonged hospitalization. In an outbreak of gastroenteritis involving a number of hospitals, salmonellosis became a special problem in patients with various tumors who were being fed egg-enriched dietary supplements contamined by *S. derby* [427,429,459]. In non-epidemic periods, *S. typhimurium* is the most common serotype isolated from all cases of acute enteritis, including those with cancer [429].

Focal infections of primary and metastatic tumors by salmonella have been observed in a number of instances [251,426–429,481–483]. These are probably the result of the deposition of the organisms in the lesions during an episode of transient bacteremia. It has been suggested that the presence of cancer of the colon predisposes to systemic invasion when salmonella invade the intestine [427,484]. This occurs most often where tumors are excised.

Patients with leukemia and lymphoma, including Hodgkin's disease, are highly susceptible to invasion of the bloodstream by salmonella [429,459,485]. This has been documented by experiences at the New York Memorial Hospital, where 35% of all cases and 74% of those with leukemia and lymphoma had bacteremia in the course of infection by this group of organisms [429]. Thirteen per cent of individuals with salmonella in the circulation have been noted to have underlying lymphoproliferative disorders [459]. *S. typhimurium* has been observed to be the most common serotype involved. Other important and unusual aspects of these infections in immunosuppressed people are (a) an increase in frequency of pleuro-pulmonary disease, (b) relatively low incidence of enteritis and the asymptomatic carrier state and (c) a very high fatality rate determined by both the basic disease and the complicating bacterial invasion [429,480].

The factors that predispose patients with neoplastic disease, especially those with lymphoproliferative disorders, to salmonellosis have not been clearly identified. Hypogammaglobulinemia does not appear to play an important role. However, impaired cellular immunity, hemolysis and leukopenia probably increase susceptibility [427,459,485]. Therapy of tumors with corticosteroids, irradiation and cytotoxic drugs may expose individuals to invasion by salmonella [427,429]. Treatment with steroids [486], alkylating agents [487] and sublethal amounts of irradiation [488] have been noted to enhance infections produced in animals by this group of organisms. These observations make it clear that every effort must be made to protect patients with neoplastic disorders, especially when they are given drugs that may produce immunosuppression, from contact with salmonella. (See Illustrative Case 17, p. 88.)

Schistosomiasis. There is a definite relation between schistosomiasis and increased susceptibility to invasion by salmonella. Although this has been noted most often in disease caused by *Schistosoma hematobium* [276,453,

454,489,490], it is also true when *S. japonicum* and *S. mansoni* [492–494] are involved. The presence of the parasitic infestation increases the frequency of persistent bacteremia and tolerance to endotoxin. The combined infection is characterized by chronic debilitating illness with loss of weight, anorexia, low grade fever and proliferation of the reticuloendothelial system similar in magnitude to that in kala-azar. This syndrome often fails to respond to therapy directed against the bacteria [276,453,454,489–494]. Five patients with chronic salmonella bacteriuria and bacteremia and urinary schistosomiasis have been described by Farid et al. [495]; high grade proteinuria and a decreased concentration of the third component of complement (C3), suggesting the presence of an immunologically mediated glomerular injury similar to that observed in typhoid fever, were also present [149]. Treatment with ampicillin eradicated the bacteria as well as the proteinuria and depression of C3 [495].

Salmonella, as well as other gram-negative bacteria, appear to have the capacity to penetrate and multiply within the schistosomes. The parasites then serve as the source for recurrent bacteremia [496,497]. Once the salmonella have invaded the schistosome they are protected both *in vitro* and *in vivo* from the effects of antibiotics [498,499]. Some chronic cases of salmonella bacteremia complicating schistosomiasis (*S. mansoni*) have been cured when therapy was directed only against the schistosome [500]. Disease of the urinary tract induced by *S. hematobium* is central to the development of chronic infection of this area by salmonella. Eradication of the bacilli depends on effective management of the anatomic defects and treatment of the schistosomiasis. Relapse of the infectious process occurs promptly when antibacterial therapy is completed, if both the structural abnormalities and the schistosomiasis have not been corrected [453,454,489,490].

Inflammatory Bowel Disease. There appears to be an increased incidence of salmonellosis in patients with any type of inflammatory disease of the bowel. Although it has been suggested that there may be a higher frequency of infection by salmonella in individuals with ulcerative colitis, statistically valid evidence for this is not presently available. Nevertheless, at least three syndromes have been described when these two diseases are associated [501–503]. Intestinal infection by the bacteria may produce a clinical, radiologic and sigmoidoscopic picture that mimics the acute inflammatory disease in all respects [257,501]. However, once the organisms have been cleared from the stool there is a complete cure of the syndrome; relapse has not been noted in a few patients who have been studied over a period of more than 15 years. The most dramatic course of events follows invasion of the bowel by members of this group of organisms when the ulcerative colitis is active. When this occurs, toxic megacolon may develop with startling rapidity and terminate in death, despite therapy with corticosteroids and total colectomy. Patients with ulcerative colitis may be carriers of various serotypes of salmonella and exhibit no ill effects. (See Illustrative cases 19, 20, 21, pp. 90, 92, 93.)

ILLUSTRATIVE CASES

Case 1

A 22 year old previously healthy white woman was admitted to the hospital with a history of fever to 103.6°F for 3 days, periumbilical pain, cramping discomfort in the right lower quadrant of the abdomen and watery diarrhea. Five days before hospitalization she had eaten barbecued chicken. Malaise, fatigue, nausea and vomiting developed 2 days later. Abdominal cramps, fever, and diarrhea appeared in the following 6 to 12 hours. Because of persistence of these symptoms and inability to eat, she sought admission to the hospital.

Physical examination revealed a pulse rate of 90 (increased to 120 on standing) and blood pressure of 110/70, without postural change. The temperature was 101.4°. Examination of the abdomen revealed moderate distension, increased bowel sounds and diffuse abdominal tenderness, particularly over the right lower quadrant. There was no organomegaly. Signs of peritonitis were absent.

Laboratory data were as follows: The hematocrit was 36.5% and white blood count 6,000/mm^3, with 50% neutrophiles, 8% bands, 29% lymphocytes, and 5% monocytes. Sedimentation rate was 31 mm/hr. Urinalysis was normal. Stool was guaiac positive, without gross blood. Gram stain of the feces revealed normal flora, and moderate numbers of polymorphonuclear leukocytes. Culture of the stool yielded *Salmonella anatum.* Cultures of blood and urine were sterile. Studies of agglutinins for salmonella were negative on the fifth day of illness and 21 days later.

Therapy consisted of intravenous administration of fluids and a glucose-rich solution of electrolytes orally as well as anti-emetics and small doses of kaopectate. Care was taken to ensure moderately hyperactive bowel sounds. Antibiotics were not given. The patient was discharged on the fifth hospital day, afebrile and feeling relatively well. Cultures of stool grew *S. anatum* 2 weeks after the onset of symptoms; they were free of this organism on culture 2, 4 and 6 weeks later.

Comment: This patient's illness represents a typical instance of gastroenteritis caused by a common offending serotype. She had ingested chicken, a food frequently contaminated with salmonella. The incubation period, type and duration of clinical manifestations and duration of carriage of the organism in the stool are characteristic of this kind of salmonellosis. The presence of blood in the feces is uncommon in adults with this kind of disease, but not unexpected. Other findings, including the presence of polymorphonuclear leukocytes in stool, a normal white blood count and failure to demonstrate an increase in agglutinins specific for *S. anatum,* are typical of the gastroenteritis produced by salmonella. The clinical management of this case exemplifies the standard practice of most physicians. Treatment consists primarily of repair of losses of fluid and electrolytes, withholding of antimicrobial agents and the use of mild antidiarrheal agents. It is important that hospital care involve strict washing of hands after contact, and sterilization of excreta. From the standpoint of protection of the health of the public, it is imperative that the proper authorities be notified.

Case 2*

A previously well 45 year old man was admitted with a 2 day history of fever without rigors, and persistent pain in the periumbilical area and right lower quadrant of the abdomen. He had not experienced nausea, vomiting, diarrhea or urinary symptoms.

Physical examination revealed a temperature of 101°F, blood pressure of 140/80, pulse 95, respirations of 18. Positive findings were restricted to the abdomen, where marked tenderness to deep palpation, with guarding and rebound tenderness, were noted in the right lower quadrant, particularly at McBurney's point. Bowel sounds were diminished. No organomegaly was noted.

At the time of admission, the hematocrit was 44%, the white blood count 7,450/mm^3, with 65% neutrophiles, 2% bands, 25% lymphocytes and 8% monocytes. A supine x-ray of the abdomen was not diagnostic.

Because of a presumptive diagnosis of acute appendicitis the patient was treated with penicillin and chloramphenicol. Exploratory laparotomy was performed and disclosed acute inflammation of the ileo-cecal area and a swollen appendix. The appendix was removed; histologic study revealed only congestion. Diarrhea ensued, fever persisted and colicky abdominal pain developed postoperatively. Stool cultures yielded *Salmonella newport.* Symptoms subsided after an additional 5 days.

Comment: This case represents an atypical presentation of gastroenteritis due to salmonella in which "classic" symptoms of appendicitis were present. If surgery had not been carried out it is very likely that all of the manifestations would have disappeared spontaneously, because they were related to an ileocolitis produced by the organism rather than to the mild edema of the appendix. The distinction between appendicitis and acute intestinal infection, on clinical grounds alone, may be very, very difficult. Because of this, it is clear that the decision to operate on this patient was justified. The typical symptoms of gastroenteritis that developed postoperatively were probably due to "activation" of a relatively quiescent infection by the surgical procedure. A large number of instances of this phenomenon have been described. In all probability, changes in the microflora induced by the antibiotics, alterations in the motility of the gut produced by anesthesia, postoperative analgesia and sur-

* Previously reported in reference 251.

gical manipulations all played an important role in "activating" the gastroenteritis in this patient. Infection of the wound and/or bacteremia, complications that may develop in surgical treatment of tissues infected by salmonella, did not occur in this case.

Case 3

A 56 year old white woman entered the hospital for an elective cholecystectomy. Eight years prior to admission she had travelled to the Far East and had experienced a prolonged episode of diarrhea, the cause of which was not elucidated. For several years prior to admission, she had been intolerant to fatty and fried foods. Two months before being hospitalized, she had been ill with nausea, vomiting, discomfort in the epigastrium and right upper quadrant of the abdomen and low-grade fever for 4 days. These symptoms subsided spontaneously. When seen one week later by her physician, gall stones were noted on abdominal x-ray. Physical examination and the results of "routine" laboratory tests were normal limits. Cholecystectomy was recommended.

Six hours after cholecystectomy and exploration of the common duct were carried out, the patient experienced a shaking chill, developed a temperature of 103°F and became hypotensive. She was treated with fluid replacement, erythromycin and chloramphenicol. Cultures of the blood and bile made at the time of operation grew a chloramphenicol-sensitive strain of *Salmonella enteritidis*. Histologic study of the gall bladder revealed chronic cholecystitis and cholelithiasis. Despite the initial stormy course, recovery occurred over a period of 10 days of antimicrobial therapy. However, culture of stool continued to yield the original strain of salmonella for 3 months after operation.

Comment: This case is an example of an unsuspected infection of the gallbladder caused by salmonella that may have had its origin in the gastroenteritis that had occurred 8 years earlier. The organisms had probably lain dormant in the gallbladder and the stones it contained over this long period. Although cultures of the stool had not been carried out preoperatively, it is very likely that the patient had been an intestinal carrier for many years as a result of continued discharge of infected bile into the gut. It is also possible that the bacteria were "hidden" within the gallstones. Although this case of cholangitis and bacteremia was caused by salmonella, an identical syndrome may be produced by any member of the *Enterobacteriaceae*. A relatively short course of antibiotics was unable to eradicate the intestinal carrier state, and may actually have prolonged the duration of carriage.

Case 4

A 51 year old man was admitted to the hospital because he had had fever, severe cramping lower abdominal pain and 15–20 loose stools per day for the preceding 72 hours. Over the 24 hours prior to hospitalization, weakness and dizziness, on attempting to arise from bed, had been a problem. The patient had undergone subtotal gastrectomy and vagotomy for severe duodenal ulcer disease 4 years earlier, and had had no difficulty until the onset of the present illness.

Physical examination at the time of admission revealed a temperature of 102°F, blood pressure of 90/60 reduced to 60/0 in the sitting position and pulse rate of 120 increasing to 150/minute when he sat up. Other positive findings were restricted to the abdomen; bowel sounds were markedly hyperactive and there was marked tenderness in the right and left lower quadrants, with moderate rebound.

The hematocrit was 50% and the white blood count 8,600/mm^3, with 60% neutrophiles, 9% bands, 28% lymphocytes and 3% monocytes. The BUN was 40 mg/dcl, creatinine 1.2 mg/dcl, sodium 153 mEq/L and potassium 2.9 mEq/L. The stools were watery, guaiac-positive and contained large numbers of polymorphonuclear leukocytes. Culture of the feces and blood yielded *Salmonella typhimurium.*

The patient was treated with large volumes of intravenous fluids and replacement of potassium. Deodorized tincture of opium was administered to moderate the marked hyperperistalsis, but severe diarrhea continued for 5 days, and then gradually resolved over the next 10 days. Ampicillin given intravenously for 3 days exacerbated the symptoms and was discontinued. Cultures of stool remained positive for two months after hospitalization.

Comment: This patient's episode of salmonellosis was characterized by a severe cholera-like syndrome resulting in hemoconcentration, hypernatremia, hypokalemia and severe compromise of the intravascular space. This type of presentation is very rare. It occurs most often in individuals with gastrectomy and its accompanying achlorhydria and rapid transit of food and pathogenic bacteria into the small intestine.

Case 5

A nine day-old white girl was admitted to the hospital with fever and progressive obtundation. She was the product of a normal pregnancy and vaginal delivery and weighed 7 lbs., 8 oz. at birth. When she left the hospital at 5 days of age she appeared entirely normal. The mother had been well throughout her pregnancy, with the exception of abdominal cramps and several loose stools for two days prior to delivery. One day prior to hospitalization the baby began to have copious diarrhea and fed poorly. The next day, her responses were noted to be relatively poor. The temperature had risen to 102°F.

Physical examination at the time of admission disclosed a slightly icteric infant, with a weak cry, a temperature of 103°F, pulse of 140 and blood pressure of 90/60. The neck was markedly stiff and the fontanelles were bulging. The liver was enlarged.

Initial laboratory studies indicated a hematocrit of 37%, and a white blood count of 3,100/mm,[3] with 42% neutrophiles, 32% bands and 26% lymphocytes. Lumbar puncture revealed an opening pressure of 260 mm H_2O. The spinal fluid contained 432 white cells, 98% of which were polymorphonuclear leukocytes. The concentrations of protein and glucose were 110 and 23 mg/dcl, respectively. Cultures of the fluid, blood and stool yielded *Salmonella heidelberg*.

Despite prompt treatment with large doses of chloramphenicol administered intravenously, the child died nine hours after she was brought to the hospital. Culture of the mother's stool grew a strain of *S. heidelberg* similar to that recovered from her baby.

Comment: This case is an example of transmission of a salmonella from a relatively asymptomatic mother to her newborn baby. Although invasion of the infant probably occurred during delivery, it might also have been related to improper precautions such as inadequate washing of the hands of the mother any time after birth of the child. The course of events in the baby suggests the initial development of gastroenteritis, followed by bacteremia and invasion of the meninges. The relatively high risk of potentially lethal complications (bacteremia and meningitis) in neonates justifies prompt treatment with antimicrobial agents such as ampicillin, amoxicillin or trimethoprim-sulfamethoxazole. The purpose of this therapy is not to cure the intestinal infection but rather to prevent the bacteremia and focal disease. In instances in which there is suspicion that maternal salmonellosis may be transmitted to infants during or after delivery, it is very important that cultures be obtained from the mother and all hospital personnel in contact with her, as well as that meticulous care of their hands be practiced. Strict isolation of infected infants and mothers is indicated while they are in hospital to forestall potential person-to-person outbreaks of infection in this susceptible group of patients.

Case 6

A 22 year old man was admitted to the hospital after he had had increasing fever, malaise, anorexia, fatigability, nonproductive cough and lower abdominal pain for 9 days. He had returned 2 weeks before the onset of symptoms from an extended trip to Nepal, where he had taken no special precautions regarding food or water. Several brief episodes of diarrhea had occurred during his travels. He had received two doses of typhoid vaccine prior to leaving the United States. The present illness began insidiously. Symptoms gradually worsened and the temperature finally reached 104°F. Although he had had a few loose stools, he was more constipated than usual, for most of the time.

At the time of entry to the hospital, the temperature was 103°F, pulse 84 and respiratory rate 18. The abdomen was distended; bowel sounds were hypoactive. The liver was enlarged (16 cm in over-all span) and the spleen was palpable 4 cm below the left costal margin. The lower abdomen was diffusely tender, especially in the right lower quadrant.

Laboratory studies revealed an hematocrit of 39%, and a white blood count of 2,600/mm^3, with 60% neutrophiles, 19% lymphocytes and 21% monocytes. The urine contained 3+ protein, 5–10 white blood cells and an occasional erythrocyte per high power field. Stool was guaiac-negative. SGOT was normal, but serum alkaline phosphatase was 2½ times higher than normal and total bilirubin was 2 mg%. Titers of agglutinating antibody for the Group D 0-antigen was 1:160, and for the H-antigen 1:120. Cultures of blood, stool, and urine grew *S. typhi.*

The patient was treated intravenously with 4 grams of chloramphenicol per day for two weeks. Symptoms began to ameliorate after 24 hours of therapy, and the temperature returned to normal after 96 hours. Titers of antibodies to the organism were unchanged after 2 weeks of treatment. The patient was discharged from the hospital on the 20th day, after being afebrile for 5 days following cessation of the administration of chloramphenicol.

Comment: This typical case of uncomplicated typhoid fever represents the disease as it is seen in the United States today. It usually occurs in individuals who return to this country after being in an area of the world where the infection is endemic. The presentation of the illness with "flu-like" symptoms, its duration, the abdominal findings, mild cholestatic jaundice, relative bradycardia, leukopenia and prompt response to chloramphenicol are all characteristic of typhoid fever. The "positive" Widal test was not diagnostic in this patient because he had received typhoid vaccine. The diagnosis rests on the isolation and identification of organisms recovered from the blood, stool or urine.

Case 7

A 46 year old man with proved typhoid fever was transferred from another hospital because of severe lower gastrointestinal bleeding. The patient had been well until 2 weeks after a skiing trip, when he and a number of other people who accompanied him developed an influenza-like syndrome with progressively rising fever and abdominal discomfort. When studied at the hospital in his community, he was found to have *S. typhi* in the bloodstream and was treated with 4 grams of chloramphenicol per day intravenously. The temperature fell and symptoms abated during the first 3 days of therapy. On the 4th day he passed a maroon-colored stool, and bleeding continued for the next 3 days. When sigmoidoscopy to 25 cm failed to reveal the source of the blood, the patient was sent to another hospital.

Physical examination on admission revealed a chronically ill appearing man with normal vital signs. The liver and spleen were enlarged. Bowel sounds were normal. The abdomen was not tender. A large reddish-colored, grossly guaiac-positive stool was passed during the physical examination.

Because of continued bleeding, exploratory laparotomy was carried out and disclosed a necrotic area (3 × 2 cm) in the ileum; a partial resection of this part of the gut was performed. Therapy with chloramphenicol, continued for an additional two weeks, led to complete recovery, without clinical or bacteriologic relapse.

Comment: Severe hemorrhage due to necrosis and sloughing of ileal mucosa continues to be a problem in patients with typhoid fever, and does not represent failure of antimicrobial therapy. Although conservative management is usually recommended when intestinal hemorrhage complicates this disease, surgery is required in some cases. The present approach to this problem involves localization of the site of bleeding by angiography, followed by the injection of Pitressin, prepared clot or Gelfoam^{R} in an attempt to control the bleeding. If this is unsuccessful, or significant rebleeding occurs, prompt surgical intervention is undertaken. Antimicrobial therapy is continued for the usual period.

Case 8

A 14 year old Mexican boy who had recently left Mexico City was sent to the hospital because he had had fever, malaise, anorexia, abdominal pain and a nonproductive cough for 6 days. Two other family members had developed similar symptoms a few days earlier. A chloramphenicol-resistant strain of *Salmonella typhi* had been isolated from their stools and blood.

Physical examination at the time of admission revealed a temperature of 103°F and pulse and respiratory rates of 85 and 20/minute, respectively. The patient appeared chronically ill and complained of abdominal pain. The abdomen was distended and diffusely tender; bowel loops were dilated and sounds were decreased. The spleen was enlarged. The liver was normal in size.

When admitted to the hospital, the patient's hematocrit was 38%, and white blood count, 3,200/mm^3, with 62% neutrophiles, 4% band forms, 18% lymphocytes and 16% monocytes. The urine was normal. Feces were free of blood. Cultures of stool and blood yielded a chloramphenicol-resistant, ampicillin-sensitive *Salmonella typhi.* The titer of agglutinating antibody for Group D 0 antigen was 1:80, and for H antigen 1:120.

Therapy with 8 gm of ampicillin/day intravenously was begun. Symptoms subsided, and the temperature began to decrease during the second day of treatment. Increasingly severe abdominal pain, especially in the right lower quadrant, appeared on the 3rd day. The temperature rose to 104°F, and tachycardia and slight hypotension developed. At this time, definite evidence of peritonitis (absent bowel sounds and marked rebound tenderness) became apparent. The white blood count was 14,000, with 72% neutrophiles, 18% band forms and 10% lymphocytes. Surgical exploration disclosed one large and several smaller perforations of a paper-thin area in the ileum, and diffuse peritonitis; the involved part of the bowel was resected. Culture of the peritoneal fluid yielded *E. coli, Klebsiella pneumoniae, Pseudomonas aeruginosa,* anaerobic streptococci, and *Bacteroides fragilis,* but not salmonella. Clindamycin and gentamicin were added to the ampicillin. Recovery was uneventful.

Comment: This is a case of typhoid fever due to chloramphenicol-resistant *S. typhi* that was acquired in Mexico City, an area in which such strains of the organism are common. Intestinal perforation occurred despite appropriate therapy with ampicillin. This represents a complication of the disease and not a failure of the chemotherapy. Several important clinical points are illustrated by the course of the patient's infection. A striking leukocytosis replaced the leukopenia characteristic of typhoid fever after intestinal perforation occurred. Failure to demonstrate *S. typhi* in the peritoneal fluid from which members of the normal microflora of the intestine were recovered is the rule. Prompt surgical therapy was probably life-saving in this patient. The levels of agglutinating antibody detected at the time of admission to the hospital are in the range of those present in persons who live in areas where typhoid fever is endemic, and were of no diagnostic value.

Case 9

A 69 year old man presented to the hospital because, for the preceding 3 months, he had experienced pain in the lower back, sweating, temperatures up to 102°F, anorexia and a loss of 25 pounds. He was a construction engineer whose occupation had taken him to most of the countries in the world. He had had malaria, bacillary dysentery, amebiasis and typhoid fever in the remote past. He had resided in the United States for the past 10 years and had no important illness during this period.

The temperature was 101°F. Percussion over the lower thoracic spine and straight leg raising produced pain. No other abnormal findings were detected. Neurologic study revealed no evidence of dysfunction.

The hematocrit was 34%, and the white blood count 7,200/mm^3, with 72% neutrophiles, 18% lymphocytes and 10% monocytes; the sedimentation rate was 88 mm/hr. The urine was normal. Serum albumin and globulin were 3.2 and 3.9 gm/dcl. Serum electrophoresis indicated a polyclonal increase in the gamma globulins. Cultures of blood and urine were sterile; stool contained no pathogenic organisms. The titers of agglutinating antibody for the group D O and H antigens of *S. typhi* were 1/640 and 1/240, respectively. Radiographic examination of the thoracic spine disclosed narrowing of the intervertebral space between D11 and 12, destruction of the surfaces of these vertebrae and a paravertebral mass (Fig. 9).

Culture of material obtained by needle biopsy of the space between D11 and 12 yielded *S. typhi*. Treatment with 12 gm/day of ampicillin given intravenously was instituted and continued for 6 weeks. The patient refused surgical drainage of the paravertebral mass. Clinical improvement became apparent after 10 days of therapy and continued. At the time of discharge from the hospital, the patient had no fever and was free of pain. The sedimentation rate had decreased to 34 mm/hr.

Comment: This patient exemplifies the ability of *S. typhi* to invade a tissue, especially bone, during an acute episode of infection, become sequestered, and, after remaining *in situ* for many years, produce active disease. The Widal test may be useful in indicating the diagnosis in such cases. However, microbiologic confirmation is necessary. Although ideal management of the patient should have involved not only antibacterial chemotherapy but also drainage of the paravertebral lesion, this was not possible. For this reason, there was a continued risk of relapse of the infection.

Case 10*

A 68 year old man was admitted to the hospital because of low grade fever, sweating, malaise, anorexia, weight loss and abdominal pain that had been present for 5 weeks. The pain was localized to the hypogastric region; it was continuous and radiated into the left groin and testis, but was unrelated to urination, defecation or position. The patient had had hypertension for many years, and had undergone bilateral lumbar sympathectomy 7 years earlier because of peripheral vascular insufficiency with intermittent claudication.

Physical examination revealed the temperature to be 101°F, the blood pressure 230/100 and the pulse 80/min. The heart was enlarged; there was a grade II/VI systolic murmur. The liver was slightly enlarged. The left flank was tender. The hematocrit was 36%, and the white blood count 10,800/mm^3, with 76% neutrophiles, 4% band forms, 13% lymphocytes and 7% monocytes. Cultures of the blood, urine and stool grew a nontyphoidal group D salmonella. Titers of agglutinating antibody for Groups B and D were high.

The patient's temperature remained at 100–102°F, and he continued to complain of moderately severe hypogastric pain and tenderness in the left flank. Treatment was initiated with 2 gm chloramphenicol per day given intravenously. Culture of blood carried out on the 3rd day of therapy was still positive for salmonella. Intravenous pyelograph on the 30th day in the hospital

* This case has been reported previously as a clinico-pathologic conference in New England Journal of Medicine 266:249–255, 1962.

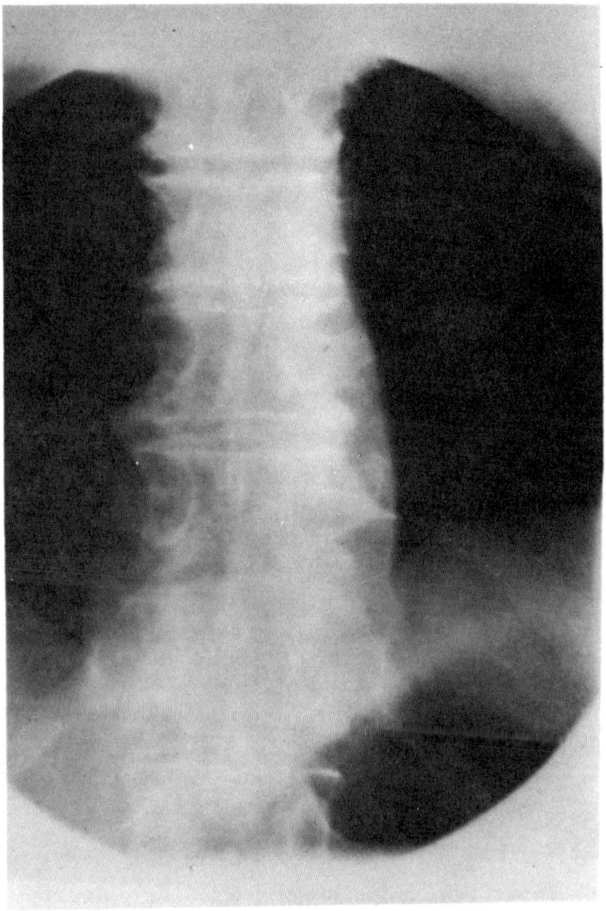

FIG. 9. X-ray of the thoracic spine of Illustrative Case 9, demonstrating narrowing of the intervertebral space between D11 and 12, destruction of the contiguous surfaces of these vertebrae, and an associated paravertebral mass. Needle biopsy of the intervertebral disc space yielded *Salmonella typhi*.

revealed a shift in the position of the left kidney and of the most lateral paravertebral metal clip applied during the sympathectomy; an earlier study of the kidneys had disclosed no abnormalities. Two days later, the patient was unable to extend the left hip, and held the left leg in flexion and external rotation. A nontender pulsatile mass with an audible bruit was detected in the left lower abdomen. There was a sudden increase in abdominal pain, accompanied by a sensation of fullness in the left flank, on the 17th day of hospitalization. Surgical exploration of the abdomen revealed a leaking "paper-thin" aneurysm of the aorta and hemorrhage and abscess in the psoas muscle (Fig. 10). The

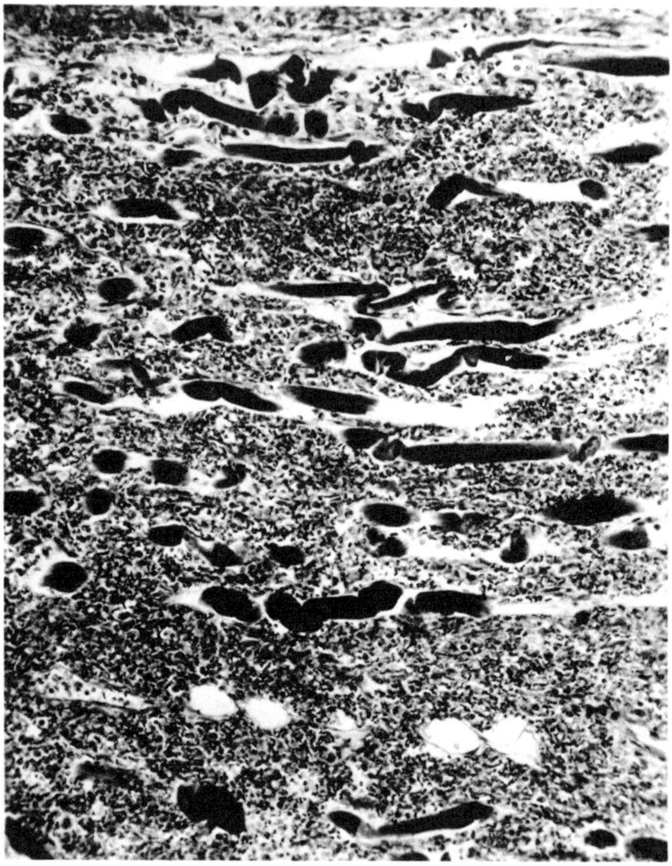

FIG. 10. High power light microscopic view of the psoas abscess due to a Group D salmonella in Illustrative Case 10. There is an intense leukocytic infiltrate widely separating the remaining darkly staining muscle fibers.

aneurysm ruptured during surgery and the patient expired. Culture of the involved area of the aorta and the abscess grew Group D salmonella.

Comment: This is a classic instance of bacteremia complicating gastroenteritis caused by salmonella resulting in infection of an atherosclerotic aorta, and the development of a mycotic aneurysm that ruptured. The possibility that this course of events may appear in elderly individuals with known vascular disease who initially experience an uncomplicated enteric infection caused by salmonella justifies treatment of the intestinal syndrome with antibiotics. The persistence of high grade bacteremia and the continuously positive blood cultures after 3 days of appropriate antimicrobial therapy should have raised a strong suspicion that the infection had metastasized to an intravascular site. Evaluation of the heart and abdominal angiography would have disclosed the aneurysm. Had this been detected and treated early, the development of the abscess in the psoas muscle and rupture of the aorta might have been prevented. A somewhat unusual feature of this case is the involvement of a group D salmonella rather than *S. choleraesuis* or *S. typhimurium,* the serotypes most commonly associated with this syndrome.

Case 11*

A 62 year old previously healthy man came to the hospital because he had had fever to 103°F, shaking chills, anorexia, malaise and a loss of 40 pounds during the preceding 10 weeks. Although he was not certain, he may have had a transient episode of diarrhea about a week prior to the onset of the present illness.

At the time of hospitalization, the temperature was 102°F, blood pressure 160/70, and the pulse 95/min. No abnormal findings were detected during physical examination.

The hematocrit was 34% and the white blood count 10,000/mm^3, with 76% neutrophiles, 22% lymphocytes and 2% monocytes. The sedimentation rate was 85 mm/hr. The urine contained 2+ protein and 5–10 white blood cells per high power field. Cultures of blood (5/10), stool and urine grew chloramphenicol- and ampicillin-sensitive *Salmonella enteritidis.* A double-dose oral cholecystogram failed to demonstrate the gallbladder.

The patient was treated intravenously with 4 gm chloramphenicol per day. However, hectic fever continued, and cultures of the blood remained positive. Because these findings suggested the possibility of an infected intravascular site, a nuclear scan (Fig. 11) and ultrasound study (Fig. 12) of the abdomen were carried out. The results of these suggested an abdominal aortic aneurysm. A transfemoral aortogram (Fig. 13) outlined this lesion. The patient was given large doses of ampicillin, and underwent resection of the aneurysm. A dacron graft from the thoracic aorta was brought extrapleurally and then extraperitoneally and anastomosed to the distal external iliac arteries, after which the abdominal aorta, from just distal to the renal arteries to the common iliac bifurcation, was removed and the aorta and iliac vessels were closed. Extensive acute and chronic inflammation were noted in the retroperitoneal bed. Cultures of this area grew *Salmonella enteritidis.* The gallbladder was removed; it was anatomically normal and sterile. Ampicillin was given intravenously for 6 weeks. Recovery was complete and uneventful.

Comment: The important point made by this case is the fact that, because of persistent bacteremia despite appropriate antimicrobial therapy, the possibility of an intravascular focus was suspected. This led to the use of diagnostic modalities that demonstrated a lesion in the aorta. Radionuclide scans and

* Previously published case, reference 272.

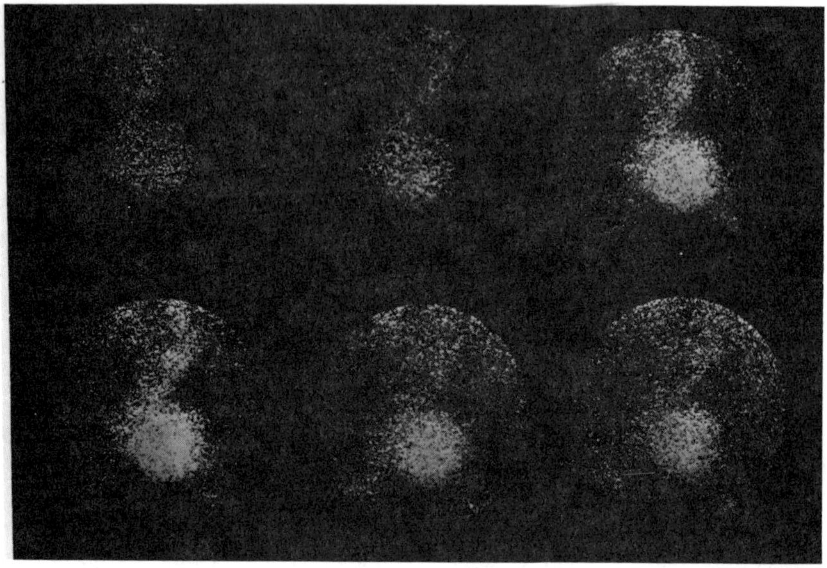

FIG. 11. Serial images in a radionuclide blood pool scan, demonstrating aneurysmal dilitation of the abdominal aorta.

ultrasound may be helpful in demonstrating the presence of an aortic aneurysm, although aortography remains the definitive diagnostic procedure. The two findings of an aneurysm and persistent bacteremia led to the diagnosis of an infected aneurysm, requiring surgical as well as medical therapy. Particularly noteworthy was the demonstration of infection in the retroperitoneal space. This is fairly common with infection of aortic aneurysms, and accounts for the high incidence of rupture of grafts when they are placed in the aorta. Although this may be successful in some instances, the safer procedure is the one carried out in this patient, in which uninfected tissue planes lie between the aortic graft and the infected retroperitoneal tissue. It is not known whether

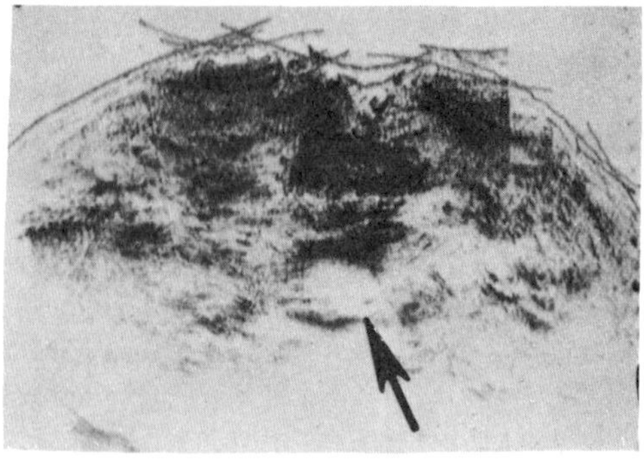

FIG. 12. Abdominal grey scale ultrasound examination, transverse view, demonstrating aneurysmal dilitation of the abdominal aorta (arrow).

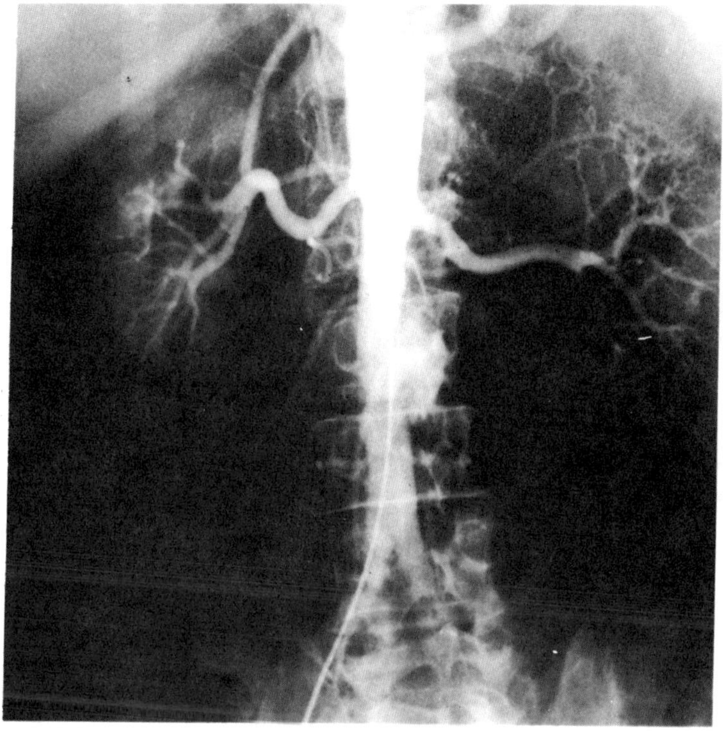

FIG. 13. Transfemoral aortogram performed on Illustrative Case 11, demonstrating a saccular mycotic aneurysm of the abdominal aorta below the level of the renal arteries.

chloramphenicol or ampicillin is the drug of choice in the management of intravascular infections caused by nontyphoidal serotypes of salmonella. Extrapolation from endocarditis and endarteritis caused by other bacteria suggests that therapy with a bactericidal (ampicillin) rather than a bacteriostatic (chloramphenicol) agent may produce better results.

Case 12

The patient was a 59 year old woman who had had intermittent episodes of bacteremia with *Salmonella javiana* for 3 months. She had old rheumatic heart disease, with mitral stenosis and well controlled atrial fibrillation, but was reasonably well until 3 months before admission to the hospital, when she and her husband developed fever, malaise, anorexia and diarrhea. Her husband's symptoms cleared. However, hers did not, and, for this reason, her blood was cultured and yielded *Salmonella javiana*. Treatment with intravenous ampicillin, cephalothin, and gentamicin led to defervescence. Three days after therapy was stopped, fever recurred and blood cultures again became positive. The patient was treated with ampicillin, carbenicillin and chloramphenicol over the next 3 months and had her gallbladder removed; no salmonella were detected in the gallstones. The temperature became elevated and bacteremia occurred each time antibiotics were discontinued or drugs were given by the oral route.

When admitted to the hospital, the patient's temperature was 102°F. Atrial fibrillation at a rate of 120 was present. She was moderately lethargic. Examination of the heart revealed an opening snap and a loud rumbling mitral diastolic murmur. The liver and spleen were slightly enlarged. Neurologic examination disclosed a mild left hemiparesis and an extensor plantar response on the same side.

The hematocrit was 35%, and the white blood count 21,000/mm^3, with 89% neutrophiles, 4% band forms, 5% monocytes and 2% eosinophiles. The urine was normal. Cultures of the blood and stool yielded *Salmonella javiana*. The cerebrospinal fluid was normal. Cerebral angiography revealed multiple emboli in the right middle or anterior cerebral arteries. Abdominal angiograms disclosed no abnormalities.

Treatment was initiated with 15, and later 18, gm ampicillin per day intravenously. Because fever and bacteremia persisted, therapy was changed to 90 million units of penicillin per day. Because this produced seizures, the daily dose was reduced to 40–60 million units. Despite this, manifestations of infection remained unaltered. For this reason, cardiac surgery was carried out in the 4th month of illness. The mitral valve was found to be stenotic and calcified, but was free of endocarditis. The left atrium contained a large, multi-pocketed, ulcerating thrombus covered with purulent exudate. Cultures of this revealed *Salmonella javiana*. The patient died a few hours after the surgical procedure was completed.

Comment: This case illustrates many of the major characteristics of endocarditis caused by salmonella. These include (a) the propensity of the organism to infect unusual cardiac sites as well as heart valves, particularly preexisting thrombi and abnormal mural surfaces, (b) the frequent, if not invariable, inability of even massive doses of effective antimicrobial agents to eradicate the infectious process, (c) the importance of surgical removal of the infected locus, and (d) the need for early consideration of surgical intervention. This kind of disease raises the important issue of chemoprophylaxis in individuals with heart disease when they develop gastroenteritis due to salmonella. Although antibiotics in individuals with valvular heart disease and salmonella gastroenteritis will not help the gastroenteritis, they may protect the abnormal heart against the consequences of a transient bacteremia. Therefore, therapy with ampicillin, amoxicillin or trimethoprim-sulfamethoxazole is recommended in such patients. This patient probably should have been operated earlier than she was, especially when it became apparent that medical therapy had no effect on the course of illness. It must be pointed out, however, that operative procedures involving the heart in patients like the one described pose considerable hazard.

Case 13

A 47 year old previously healthy woman came to the hospital because she had had fever, malaise and a swollen tender right breast for 3 days. She had no unusual travel or food exposure. There was no recent trauma to the involved breast.

At the time of hospitalization, the temperature was 101°F. The right breast was swollen. A tender area of induration about 5 × 3 cm in size was noted; the skin over it was erythematous. The left breast and the remainder of the physical examination were within normal limits.

The hematocrit was 40%, and the white blood count 15,000/mm^3, with 60% neutrophiles, 10% band forms and 5% monocytes. Cultures of blood were sterile. Agglutinins for salmonella were not detected. Culture of stool revealed no enteric pathogens. The lesion in the breast was drained surgically. About 150 ml of creamy, nonfoul pus were evacuated; cultures of this grew *Salmonella choleraesuis.* Treatment with ampicillin given intravenously was carried out for 2 weeks and led to uneventful recovery.

Comment: This case is an example of infection of soft tissue by the serotype of salmonella most likely to cause metastatic focal disease. As in most instances of infection produced by this species, the patient had not had any gastrointestinal disturbances and the organism was not present in the feces. Outside of the cardiovascular and reticuloendothelial systems and the skeleton, the breast is probably the commonest area of focalization of salmonella. Combined medical and surgical therapy usually cures the mastitis without difficulty.

Case 14

A 23 year old man was admitted to the hospital with a history of 3 days of low grade fever, dysuria, urgency, suprapubic discomfort and scrotal tenderness and swelling. During the preceding two months, he had spent a great deal of time camping in Jamaica, where he ate native food, including goat intestine, and in Cape Cod, and Maine where he consumed raw roots and berries gathered in swampy areas. One month before he came to the hospital, he began to have fever, malaise, anorexia and headache; dysuria, hematuria, urgency and pain in the lower back appeared the next day. Medical evaluation at that time revealed evidence of prostatitis and right-sided epididymitis. Culture of urine, after prostatic massage, and of stool grew *Salmonella uzaramo* sensitive to all antibiotics active against most gram-negative bacteria. Symptoms disappeared after treatment with ampicillin orally for 2 weeks. Culture of the urine following cessation of therapy failed to grow salmonella. The patient remained well until 3 days prior to entry to the hospital when, after he had spent an afternoon diving, he developed increasing scrotal and suprapubic discomfort, dysuria and a temperature of 100°F.

The only abnormalities detected on physical examination were an enlarged, boggy, tender prostate, and swelling and tenderness of the scrotum and epidydimis.

The hematocrit was 38%, and the white blood count 8,300/mm^3, with 66% neutrophiles, 13% lymphocytes and 20% monocytes. Urinalysis was negative. Agglutinating titers were zero for group B 0 antigen, 1/80 for group C and 1/20 for Group D. When retitrated 5 days later, the values were 1/40 for group B, 1/640 for group C and 1/320 for group D. Cultures of urine and blood were sterile. *Salmonella uzaramo* (a Group C organism) was recovered from the feces.

Treatment with 8 gm/day of ampicillin given intravenously was initiated. Because the response over the first 10 days of therapy was slow, the patient was given sulfamethoxazole-trimethoprim for 3 months. Cultures of stool grew the salmonella for 2 months after discharge from the hospital. The patient was known to be well 8 months after therapy was completed.

Comment: The source of the unusual serotype of salmonella that infected this patient was probably goat intestine that he had eaten in Jamaica. The disease appears to have started with gastroenteritis, and was complicated by bacteremia with focalization in the genitourinary tract. A short course of antimicrobial therapy suppressed but did not eradicate the infection which had become established in the prostate. It is probable that the trauma associated with prolonged diving activated the latent focus in this organ, and produced acute prostatitis and epidydimitis. Trimethoprim-sulfamethoxazole appears to be optimal treatment for this kind of disease because the preparation is highly active against salmonella, and because the trimethoprim penetrates the prostate. The titers of agglutinating antibody detected in the patient are interesting. The greater than four-fold increase in antibody for the Group C somatic antigen is very suggestive of infection by a member of this group of salmonella. However, care must be exercised in the evaluation of such data. An equal rise in "diagnostic titer" occurs in instances of inflammation unrelated to invasion by salmonella; among such disorders are subacute bacterial endocarditis and chronic active hepatitis. The increase in titer of agglutinin for the somatic antigens of other groups of salmonella is an example of the "crossover" that may occur. It is clear that, although the results of serologic studies may be suggestive, establishment of the diagnosis rests solidly on isolation and identification of the salmonella involved.

Case 15

A 15 year old girl was admitted to the hospital complaining of fever and painful swelling over the left buttock. She had been in good health until 3 weeks earlier, when, while on a camping trip to Canada, she was struck by an automobile and sustained fractures of the right fibula and left sacrum. The leg was placed in a cast. A large hematoma developed over the buttock. Two hundred ml of blood was evacuated from this area after one week, and an additional 100 ml 3 days later. For 3 days prior to her second hospitalization, the temperature was 102°F and she complained of malaise and anorexia.

The only important physical findings when she was admitted were a temperature of 101°F, a cast on the right leg and a large tender hematoma over the left buttock.

The hematocrit was 34%, and the white blood count 20,000, with 81% neutrophiles, 4% band forms, 4% lymphocytes, 9% monocytes and 2% eosinophiles. The urine was normal. Cultures of the blood and urine were negative. The hematoma was evacuated of about 250 ml of dried old blood. Cultures of this and stool grew *Salmonella newport.* Treatment with chloramphenicol intravenously was instituted and continued for 3 weeks. Defervescence occurred promptly and recovery was uneventful.

Comment: This unusual instance of soft tissue infection by *Salmonella newport* probably represents a complication of an asymptomatic episode of gastroenteritis due to this organism. It is most likely that contamination of the skin over the buttock by salmonella present in the intestinal tract led to inoculation of the hematoma when it was drained. Although a transient bacteremia, with focalization into the area of hemorrhage might have been involved, this does not appear to be as likely a possibility.

Case 16

A 65 year old man was admitted to the hospital for evaluation of severe pain that had been present over the right lower leg for 10 days. This was an exacerbation of a sensation of aching in the same area that had been present for the preceding 5 months. There had been no fever or manifestations of gastrointestinal dysfunction. The only abnormality detected on physical examination was a warm, tender, oval-shaped area, 3 × 5 cm in size, at the junction of the middle and lower third of the right tibia.

The hematocrit was 48.7%. The white blood count was 10,200/mm^3, with 73% neutrophiles, 21% lymphocytes, and 5% monocytes. The sedimentation rate was 11 mm/hr. Tomographic studies of the tibia disclosed an irregular lytic area, and marked endosteal response in the middle of the bone. Bone scan revealed increased activity in the same site. Multiple cultures of blood, urine, and stool were negative. The titers of agglutinating antibody for salmonella were 1/160, 1/320 and zero for groups B, C and D, respectively.

Because it was not possible to decide whether the tibial lesion was osteomyelitis or a tumor, biopsy was carried out. Cultures of the biopsied tissue were sterile, but the histologic findings were consistent with chronic osteomyelitis. A second titration for agglutinating antibody for salmonella revealed that it had increased from 1/320 to 1/1280, a "diagnostic" rise, for group C organisms; titers for the other groups were unchanged. In spite of failure to recover bacteria from the bone, the patient was treated for 4 weeks with chloramphenicol and clindamycin. He appeared to improve and was discharged from the hospital. He was readmitted 2 months later because a mass had appeared at the site of the biopsy. This was removed and proved to be reticulum cell sarcoma; there was no evidence of infection, although an inflammatory reaction was present. Radiation therapy produced a good result.

Comment: This case is an excellent example of falsely positive "diagnostic" changes in titers of agglutinating antibody for salmonella. The presence of inflammatory cells in bone involved with tumor, in the absence of infection, is not unusual. It is clear that at no time did this patient have osteomyelitis due to salmonella or any other organism.

Case 17

A 59 year old man came to the hospital after he had experienced fever and shaking chills for 2 days. He had undergone successful transplantation of a kidney from a cadaver 18 months previously because of chronic renal failure secondary to diabetic nephropathy. He remained in good health while being treated with 125 mg/day of azothioprine, 20 mg/day of prednisone, and insulin. The serum creatinine was stable at 1.2 mg/dcl and the BUN at 28 mg/dcl.

Physical examination disclosed a severely ill man with cushingoid facies, a temperature of 102°F, a pulse rate of 110 and respiratory rate of 24. The heart was enlarged and there was a Grade II/VI systolic ejection murmur. There was moderate tenderness over the transplanted kidney. The prostate was enlarged and slightly tender. The hematocrit was 36%, and the white blood count 6,200/mm^3, with 70% neutrophiles, 11% band forms, 15% lymphocytes and 4% monocytes. The urine contained large numbers of polymorphonuclear leukocytes and gram-negative bacilli.

Because of evidence of infection of the urinary tract, therapy with ampicillin intravenously was started. Cultures of urine, blood and subsequently of stool grew *Salmonella typhimurium.* The chemotherapy was continued for 2 weeks and led to prompt defervescence and clearing of the urine. After discharge from the hospital, the patient was treated with trimethoprim-sulfamethoxazole for 3 months. He remained well over this period; cultures of the stool were negative during this time. One month after discontinuing cotrimoxazole, fever, chills and dysuria developed and he was readmitted to the hospital, where *S. typhimurium* was again recovered from the blood and urine despite the administration of large doses of ampicillin intravenously for a few days. A faint murmur of aortic insufficiency was heard, and there was evidence of mild congestive heart failure. Cardiac fluoroscopy revealed a calcified aortic valve.

Echocardiography confirmed this finding and, in addition, suggested a vegetation on the heart valve. Treatment with large doses of ampicillin intravenously was continued for 6 weeks. He made a good response to this therapy and was discharged from the hospital on a regimen of 2 gm/day of ampicillin to be taken orally. He is still being followed, and remains well 6 months after leaving the hospital.

Comment: Although statistically-valid data are not presently available, it is the general impression that patients with transplanted kidneys are highly susceptible to invasion by salmonella, especially metastatic infection of the urinary tract, that is difficult to eradicate. This has also been our experience. This patient is an excellent example of this phenomenon; relapsing infection of the urinary tract due to *Salmonella typhimurium* was his primary problem. However, in his case, focalization of the organism also involved a previously abnormal aortic valve. Under usual circumstances, optimal therapy would have included replacement of the affected valve early in the course of the disease, in addition to appropriate antimicrobial therapy. Severe disease of the coronary arteries, unstable diabetes mellitus, and the presence of a transplanted kidney contraindicated surgical therapy. Although the patient has continued to remain well while taking "suppressive" doses of ampicillin orally, there is a good possibility of relapse of the infection when this is discontinued.

Case 18

An 11 year old boy with known sickle cell anemia was admitted to the hospital because of fever and an exquisitely painful right thigh that had been of 3 day's duration. He had been hospitalized 3 weeks earlier for management of a sickle cell crisis featured by severe pain in the right upper leg and ribs. He also had an "upset stomach." He was treated with antipyretic and analgesic agents, hydrated and transfused; all symptoms disappeared in 5 days. There were no further problems until 3 days before the hospitalization for fever and recurrence of pain in the thigh.

Physical examination revealed a small black male whose temperature was 101°F, and who complained of severe pain when the right thigh was moved or palpated. The tip of the spleen was barely palpable. The hematocrit was 21%. The white blood count was 19,000/mm^3, with 56% neutrophiles, 14% band forms and 30% lymphocytes. The red blood cells exhibited sickling. Cultures of stool and urine were negative. Titers of agglutinating antibody for the 0 antigens of salmonella were 1/80 for group B, 1/40 for group C and 1/120 for group D. When these studies were repeated a week later, the titer for group B antigen had increased to 1/320. One of 4 cultures of the blood grew *Salmonella typhimurium* sensitive to ampicillin. Radiographic examination of the right femur demonstrated osteopenia, but no clear-cut evidence of osteomyelitis. The patient was treated with ampicillin by the intravenous route for 4 weeks.

Marked improvement was apparent after 5 days, and fever disappeared after 11 days of therapy.

Comment: This is a typical instance of osteomyelitis in a patient with sickle cell anemia, presumably as a complication of an episode of gastroenteritis 3 weeks earlier. As is often the case, the site of involvement of bone was the same as that in which a sterile infarct probably developed during the preceding sickle crisis. The absence of the typical radiographic changes of osteomyelitis is not surprising since the study was carried out early in the course of the disease. Although titration of specific antibodies may be helpful in diagnosis, falsely positive and negative results may pose a problem. Despite the appropriate chemotherapy received by the patient, he is still at risk of recurrent invasion by salmonella.

Case 19

A 24 year old woman was admitted to the hospital because she had had cramping pain in the periumbilical area and right lower quadrant, diarrhea, and fever for the preceding 6 days. The illness was ushered in by nausea and vomiting, which were followed rapidly by the appearance of abdominal pain and diarrhea. She had been passing 10–15 liquid or semi-formed stools a day; all contained large quantities of mucus; blood was noted occasionally. Past medical history was unremarkable for any type of gastrointestinal disorder.

Physical examination when the patient entered the hospital disclosed a moderately tender and distended abdomen; bowel sounds were increased. There were no signs of peritoneal irritation. The rectum was diffusely tender. Stool was guaiac positive. The temperature was 100°F. The white blood count was 6,000/mm^3, with 76% neutrophiles, 19% lymphocytes. The hematocrit was 39%.

Sigmoidoscopy disclosed a diffusely friable mucosa, without ulcerations. Gram stain of feces revealed the usual mixture of gram-positive and -negative organisms and large numbers of polymorphonuclear leukocytes. Barium enema disclosed an ahaustral left colon and accentuated irregular haustrations of the transverse colon, findings compatible with ulcerative colitis (Fig. 14). Cultures of the feces yielded a strain of *Salmonella typhimurium* resistant to ampicillin.

The patient was treated initially with prednisone 60 mg/day. Chloramphenicol was added when the results of the cultures of stool became available. All symptoms cleared rapidly. Excretion of the salmonella in the feces continued for 2 months. The dose of corticosteroid was gradually reduced and it was discontinued after 4 weeks. Sigmoidoscopy one month after the initial examination showed minimal mucosal edema; this was gone one month later. Barium enema performed 3 months after the onset of illness was normal save for a few small ulcerations.

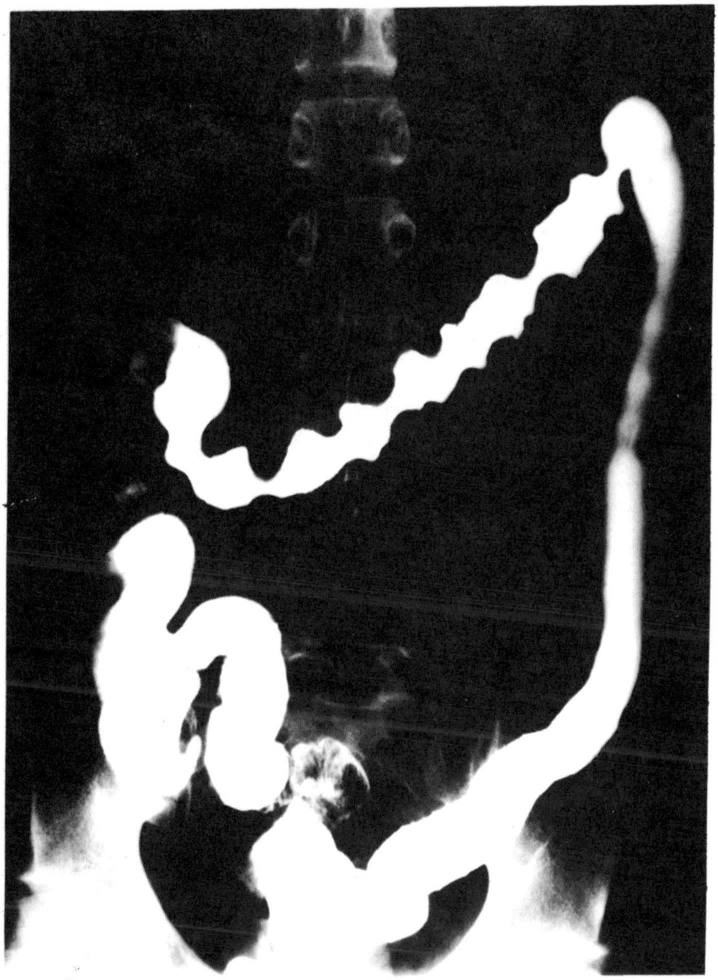

FIG. 14. Barium enema examination disclosing an ahuastral left colon, accentuated irregular haustrations in the transverse colon, and a patulous ileocecal valve.

Comment: The initial diagnosis made in this case was acute idiopathic ulcerative colitis. However, when the results of cultures of stool became available, two possibilities were considered; (a) ulcerative colitis due to salmonella, or (b) ulcerative colitis complicated by salmonellosis. Although the patient improved rapidly when given appropriate antimicrobial therapy, this might also have been related to the administration of prednisone. Although the severe degree of colonic involvement is unusual in infection of the intestine by salmonella, it may occur.

The course of events in this case makes it impossible to determine whether this was an instance of ulcerative colitis with the salmonella carrier state, ulcerative colitis produced by the organism alone, or ulcerative colitis with superimposed enteritis due to salmonella.

It has been suggested that ulcerative colitis is associated with an increased susceptibility to invasion by salmonella, and that there is a higher incidence of bacteremia in these cases. It is clear that it is difficult to distinguish these syndromes since microbiologic, cellular, sigmoidoscopic and radiologic findings may be the same at the time of presentation. Careful clinical follow-up over a prolonged time period, particularly with serial barium enema examinations, should allow one to make a judgment as to the pathophysiology involved. From a practical standpoint, however, recovery of salmonella from stool in such a patient should indicate treatment with an effective antimicrobial agent. The presence of these organisms in the blood makes antibacterial therapy mandatory.

Case 20

The patient was a 34 year old woman who had been in excellent health until 3 weeks before she was hospitalized. Her illness began about 18 hours after she had eaten a meal in a restaurant; a number of her friends had taken the same food. The patient, as well as some of her companions, developed fever, abdominal pain and diarrhea from 16 to 20 hours after they had eaten together. Although the other persons recovered from all symptoms in 24 to 72 hours, she continued to have diarrhea (6 to 8 loose stools a day), diffuse abdominal cramps and a temperature that ranged from 101 to 102 daily. After a week, she noted blood in the feces, at first in small quantities and then more prominent. She was seen by her family physician who treated her with paregoric. About 2 weeks after the onset of the disease, a barium study of the colon was carried out. Although the results were difficult to interpret, the impression was that there were no abnormalities. Because of the persistence of all the symptoms, the possibility of idiopathic ulcerative colitis was raised and she was admitted to the hospital. The patient had had no problem with diarrhea prior to onset of the present illness.

The temperature was 101.8°F; other vital signs were within normal limits. The abdo udn was digfusely tender and moderately distended; no organs or masses were palpable.

The hematocrit was 34%. The white blood count was 13,800/mm^3, with 82% polymorphonuclear leukocytes, 13% lymphocytes and 5% monocytes. Examination of the stool disclosed gross blood and large numbers of neutrophiles; gram-stained smear showed a nondiagnostic population of gram-positive and -negative bacteria, but no amebae. Cultures of feces yielded a group C salmonella on 3 separate occasions.

Sigmoidoscopic examination of the colon and rectum revealed a granular and friable mucosa and multiple ulcerations. The descending and sigmoid colon showed mucosal irregularity when studied radiographically.

Although it was not possible, on the basis of the available information, to distinguish between idiopathic ulcerative colitis, salmonella enteritis or a combination of both, it was decided to first treat for the possibility of salmonellosis. The patient was given 3 gm/day of chloramphenicol intravenously for 2 weeks. Defervescence occurred after 48 hours and diarrhea stopped after 72 hours. Sigmoidoscopy was repeated 96 hours after cessation of the chemotherapy and disclosed no ulcers and only slight granularity of the colonic mucosa. This examination was repeated each year for the next 5 years and, on each occasion, showed completely normal bowel.

Comment: This case is an example of gastroenteritis caused by salmonella progressing to a syndrome that, on the basis of clinical, sigmoidoscopic and radiologic criteria, was indistinguishable from idiopathic ulcerative colitis. It emphasizes the well known observation that diarrhea that persists for longer than one week is usually due to a cause other than salmonella or, if related to this group of organisms, represents a complication. The diagnostic dilemma presented by patients such as this one is obvious. The lesson to be learned is that demonstration of an enteric pathogen, bacteria or amebae, in individuals with the diagnostic criteria for idiopathic ulcerative colitis should first indicate treatment with drugs active against the organism. If this fails, despite eradication of the organism, conventional therapy for etiologically undefined inflammatory disease should then be undertaken.

Case 21

A 23 year old man with known idiopathic ulcerative colitis for about 4 years had been free of important manifestations until about 2 weeks before he was admitted to a hospital because of recurrence of fever, abdominal pain and moderately severe bloody diarrhea. Prior to the onset of the present illness, his disease had been well controlled by treatment with prednisone. Sigmoidoscopic and radiographic examination disclosed findings consistent with a relapse of ulcerative colitis. Cultures of the stool grew *S. schottmulleri.* Because it could not be determined whether the "relapse" was related to the chronic inflammatory disease of the bowel, or represented an unrelated episode of gastroenteritis due to salmonella, he was sent to another hospital.

On admission, the temperature was 103.2°F. Blood pressure was 112/74. Inspection revealed a severely ill, somewhat pale young man who complained of diffuse abdominal cramps. The abdomen was moderately distended and diffusely tender, without rebound.

The hematocrit was 33%, and the white blood count of 16,000, with 86% neutrophiles, 6% band forms and 14% lymphocytes. The sedimentation rate was 38 mm/hr. Examination of the stool revealed it to be watery, and to contain gross blood and very large numbers of polymorphonuclear leukocytes. Cultures of feces confirmed the presence of *S. schottmulleri*.

Sigmoidoscopic examination disclosed a very friable, bleeding rectal and colonic mucosa with multiple large and small ulcers. The findings revealed by barium enema were consistent with acute and chronic ulcerative colitis.

Treatment with chloramphenicol, 4 gm/day intravenously, was initiated. The dose of prednisone, previously 20 mg/day, was increased to 80 mg/day. Despite this, the patient's temperature remained high, abdominal pain persisted, distension became more pronounced and bloody diarrhea continued. Two days after therapy was started, it became evident that toxic megacolon had developed. Preparations were in progress for total colectomy when the patient died. Permission for autopsy was refused.

Comment: This case probably represents an instance of relapse of well controlled idiopathic ulcerative colitis induced by a superimposed infection caused by salmonella. Although cultures of the stool were not obtained prior to death, and it is, therefore, not known whether the organisms were eradicated by the antibiotic, it is very likely that, because of the relatively short duration of treatment, this had not been accomplished. The failure of response to the antibacterial drug, together with prednisone, suggests that the inflammatory disease of the bowel was exaggerated by the bacterial infection, and progressed inexorably to the development of toxic megacolon and death.

CHAPTER V

The Management of Infections Caused by Salmonella

Although it had been suggested somewhat earlier that penicillin G might be of some value, Woodward, Smadel and their colleagues, in 1948, were the first to accomplish the cure of typhoid fever, by giving chloramphenicol [504]. It is now appreciated that the successful management of this disease, and disease caused by other salmonella, requires a thorough understanding of (a) the potential usefulness of various antimicrobial agents against salmonella, (b) the problem of episomally mediated drug resistance among the salmonella, (c) the necessity of specific approaches to the management of the different syndromes associated with the general phenomenon of salmonellosis, (d) the principles of control of fluid and electrolyte balances, (e) the indications for diagnostic angiographic and noninvasive studies of the cardiovascular system and (f) the proper place and time for surgical intervention.

GENERAL PRINCIPLES

Determination of the susceptibility of an organism recovered from an infectious process to various antimicrobial agents is the basis for the selection and application of effective therapy, in most instances. However, this is not always the case when members of the genus *Salmonella* are involved because of an incomplete correlation between *in vitro* sensitivity and clinical effects. *Resistance to a drug in vitro is directly related to clinical failure, but susceptibility of a serotype, as indicated in the laboratory, does not always ensure a satisfactory therapeutic response.* For example, while the tetracycline compounds [505], polymyxins [505,506], paromomycin [506], cephalosporins [506–509], streptomycin [505], kanamycin [510,511], gentamicin [506], nalidixic acid [506] and oxolinic acid [512] all produce inhibition of growth of most strains of the organisms *in vitro*, they are virtually ineffective *in vivo*.

Only four antimicrobial agents are presently known to be effective in the treatment of infections caused by salmonella. These are *chloramphenicol* [504,505,513–515], *ampicillin* [514–521], *amoxicillin* [522–526], and the combination of *trimethoprim with sulfamethoxazole* [527–540]. In disease produced by sensitive serotypes, the therapeutic effect of chloramphenicol is the standard against which the effectiveness of other antibacterial compounds is measured. It must be administered either orally or intravenously because it is inadequately absorbed after intramuscular injection [519,541]. Comparison of the effects of small doses of ampicillin (less than 6 gm/day) with those of chloramphenicol has indicated the superiority of the latter in typhoid fever [514–521]. The comparative activity of these drugs when 8 to 12 gm of the ampicillin is administered intravenously has not been examined. Amoxicillin, a congener of ampicillin, is of value only for oral therapy of infections caused by salmonella sensitive to ampicillin. The primary advantages of this agent are higher blood levels and a lower incidence of diarrhea than follow the use of the parent compound. Trimethoprim and sulfamethoxazole, when combined, act synergistically to inhibit strains of salmonella susceptible to both drugs alone; organisms resistant to the sulfonamide may be suppressed by the trimethoprim alone [525]. Amoxicillin and the combination of sulfamethoxazole and trimethoprim are presently employed chiefly as alternate therapy for strains of salmonella resistant to other antimicrobial agents, and for oral administration to patients treated out of the hospital.

A basic assumption in the clinical management of bacterial infections has been that the use of appropriate antibiotics increases the rapidity and frequency of recovery. It is clear that this is only partially true for disease caused by salmonella. Some syndromes of salmonellosis are benefited by antimicrobial therapy, while others may actually be prolonged when exposed to these drugs. However, antibiotics may be of value in the latter when the risk of metastatic infection outweighs the potential problems associated with prolongation of illness. It is eminently clear that the different syndromes of salmonellosis require specific approaches to management if therapeutic success is to be achieved.

GASTROENTERITIS

The primary approaches to successful management of gastroenteritis due to salmonella are (a) repair of disturbances of balance of fluids and electrolytes, (b) control of symptoms such as abdominal pain, and (c) administration of appropriate antimicrobial therapy, when indicated.

A number of antibiotics, including paromomycin [542], neomycin [543], neomycin plus ampicillin [544], chloramphenicol [60,545,546], ampicillin [536,545–548] and trimethoprim-sulfamethoxazole [534,536,539,548], have been used to treat this disease. *All have failed to alter the rate of clinical recovery, and all appear to increase the incidence and duration of intestinal carriage of the organisms* [545,546,549]. It is evident, therefore, that the routine use of antibiotics in patients with acute gastroenteritis caused by salmonella is contraindicated, in most instances. There are, however, a *few* situations in which treatment with antibacterial drugs is indicated. Among these are cases in which there is an established bacteremia, or the risk of the development of this complication is high; in the latter, the drugs are given prophylactically, despite the adverse effects that may be associated with their use. Patients to be considered for such prophylaxis are (a) neonates and elderly individuals, the former because of the higher rate of bacteremia and metastatic infection, particularly meningitis, and the latter because of the risk of invasion of atherosclerotic plaques or aneurysms; (b) those with lymphoproliferative disorders, because they tolerate the presence of organisms in the bloodstream poorly [429,459,485]; (c) those with known or suspected abnormalities of the cardiovascular system, such as prosthetic heart valves, vascular grafts, aneurysms or arteriovenous malformations or rheumatic or congenital heart disease, the treatment of metastatic foci being difficult and the outcome unpredictable in these patients; (d) those with significant disorders of bones or joints and those with foreign bodies (plates, screws or rods in bone, and protheses in joints) in their skeletal systems; and (e) those with anemias featured by episodes of acute hemolysis, especially sickle cell disease. Whether or not individuals with schistosomiasis and those with preexisting inflammatory disease of the bowel might also benefit from chemoprophylaxis is unknown. In cases in which the decision to treat with an antimicrobial agent is made, the choice of drug and its dose are those generally recommended for use when bacteremia is present; therapy for 2 weeks appears to be adequate, in most instances.

The reasons for failure of antimicrobial therapy to produce early cure of gastroenteritis caused by salmonella have not been specifically identified. Dixon has hypothesized that antibiotic-induced changes in the indigenous intestinal microflora may play a role in perpetuating the infection [546]. As previously discussed (Chapter III), antibacterial drugs given prior to invasion appear to increase markedly the susceptibility to involvement by salmonella [169–175]. It is possible that alterations in the microbial population of the bowel induced by antibiotics administered after disease has started may also be of some importance; Mandell and Hook [550] have speculated that penicillinase elaborated by the autochthonous microflora may destroy administered ampicillin and lead to failure of therapy. It has been suggested that rifampin may be effective for the management of gastroenteritis caused by salmonella [551]. The activity of this drug in this situation may be related to its ability to penetrate macrophages, cells in which these organisms, as well as tubercle bacilli, are situated. This is consistent with the hypothesis that failure to respond to chemotherapy is probably related to the inability of many of the antibiotics to diffuse intracellularly. However, until this preliminary report of the efficacy of rifampicin is confirmed, antimicrobial therapy should be withheld in cases of acute gastroenteritis except in patients who are at high risk of or have already developed bacteremia.

Proper management of the balance of fluid and electrolytes is important in all patients with acute gastroenteritis due to salmonella, but is critical in young children and elderly individuals, many of whom develop the choleric or dysenteric forms of the disease [249,250]. Because the diarrheal fluid characteristic of this infection is rich in sodium, potassium and chloride, and contains moderate concentrations of protein (Chapter III), treatment is directed to the replacement of these components and correction of deficits of volume of fluid; this is readily accomplished by the intravenous administration of water and the required cations and anions. In areas of the world where parenteral therapy is unavailable, replacement of fluid and electrolytes may be accomplished by the oral route. Because glucose-facilitated absorption of glucose appears to be unaffected in gastroenteritis induced by salmonella [153], solutions of electrolytes containing glucose given by mouth may be effective in correcting losses of fluid and electrolytes. This is similar to the situation in cholera, where the glucose-facilitated absorption of sodium by the gut is also unaffected, despite the severe secretory diarrhea engendered by the toxin elaborated by the organism; glucose and electrolytes administered orally are highly effective in this disease [552–560].

Although most physicians administer a variety of agents for the relief of the abdominal pain and diarrhea associated with the gastroenteritis produced by salmonella, it must be emphasized that the increased intestinal motility responsible for these symptoms is an important defense mechanism that clears the bowel of noxious substances. Bacteremia and systemic involvement have been noted occasionally when opiates and other agents that decrease transit time in the bowel have been given. Mild relief of symptoms with such drugs as Lo-Motil® is reasonable, but attempts to completely abolish them may lead to ileus and is to be avoided. It is possible that prostaglandin synthetase inhibitors such as indomethacin may provide a more physiologic approach to the control of the discomfort [158,159]. Such therapy is still experimental.

ENTERIC FEVERS

The two major considerations in the management of the enteric fevers are (a) the choice of an appropriate antibacterial drug, and (b) the potential need for surgical intervention. The other aspects of therapy are the same as those employed in the control of any severe systemic disease. These include (a) adequate intake of calories, with consideration of intravenous hyperalimentation in patients unable to take food by mouth, despite eradication of the bacteremia;

(b) repair of imbalances of fluid and electrolytes associated with the diarrhea; (c) transfusion of blood and correction of defects in the mechanisms of clotting, when indicated; (d) administration of antipyretic agents when hyperpyrexia supervenes. The use of corticosteroids has been recommended for severely ill patients [26,505,513,561]. There is little convincing evidence, however, that these agents produce more than symptomatic relief. The present authors do not give these drugs because the potential complications that may follow their administration appear to outweigh any documented benefit.

The cornerstone of therapy of the enteric fevers is chloramphenicol [504,513,526]. Two therapeutic regimens have been employed with apparently equal success. One involves oral administration of a "loading" dose of 3 gm or 50 mg/kg followed by the same dose every 24 hours continuously, for two periods of 5 days each, interrupted by a few days of no treatment [513]. We are strongly opposed to this approach for two reasons. First, there is no valid evidence that interruption of therapy reduces the risk of recurrence of typhoid fever, the hypothesis on which this regimen is based. Second, available data indicate that practically all cases of aplasia of the bone marrow, a complication with a very high fatality rate, have been observed only in patients who have taken the drug by mouth [562]. Because of this, we prefer to administer this antibiotic only intravenously, giving 4 gm/day for 3 to 4 weeks. As pointed out earlier, the intramuscular route of administration of the succinate ester of chloramphenicol is of little or no value because of its slow rate of hydrolysis to the active compound [519,541]. All individuals receiving this agent parenterally should have a white blood count and differential, level of hemoglobin and platelet count determined no less often than every other day. Anemia, with absence of reticulocytes, is universally present. Leukopenia is much less common, and thrombopenia occurs infrequently. All of these are dose-related toxic effects of the drug, are not produced by the mechanism (unknown) responsible for aplasia of the bone marrow, and are usually reversed within 7 to 10 days after treatment is stopped. Therapy should be discontinued when the while blood count falls to 3,000/mm^3, neutrophiles are decreased to 40% or platelets reach 100,000/mm^3. Fever may increase and systemic symptoms become more marked for a short period after treatment is started.

Intestinal perforation or hemorrhage may occur despite control of the infectious process by chloramphenicol. The incidence of the chronic carrier state appears not to be reduced by treatment of typhoid and paratyphoid fevers with this drug. The relapse rate is 20% in chloramphenicol-treated cases; this is twice as high as that observed in untreated patients. The risk of death has been reduced from 12 to <5%, even in underdeveloped areas of the world; morbidity has also been markedly decreased [513].

Extensive clinical trials of the treatment of the enteric fevers with ampicillin in doses of 100 mg/kg/day (in 4 divided doses, given chiefly orally, but also intramuscularly) have indicated the following: (a) fever is present for 2 or 3 days longer than when chloramphenicol is administered; (b) as many as 10% of patients fail to respond to the drug, despite sensitivity (*in vitro*) of the causative organism; (c) the incidence of relapse and carrier state are not reduced, when compared to untreated cases [24,517–521]. Whether or not doses of ampicillin in the range of 8 to 12 gm/day intravenously might produce greater therapeutic effectiveness has not been determined. Our present practice is to restrict the use of this antibiotic to the following situations: (a) infection produced by chloramphenicol-resistant, ampicillin-sensitive organisms; (b) individuals only moderately ill and in whom large doses of the antibiotic can be administered intravenously without difficulty over the required period of therapy. When the disease increases in severity, complications appear, or relapse occurs, therapy is changed to chloramphenicol. The development of specific antibody for the organisms responsible for a given episode of enteric fever is impaired by exposure to therapeutic doses of either ampicillin or chloramphenicol [563]. Although most studies of therapy have involved patients with typhoid fever, the data that have been obtained are also applicable to enteric fever produced by other serotypes of salmonella [520].

Amoxicillin, a congener of ampicillin that differs only in the addition of a hydroxyl group at the para position of the benzene ring in the side chain of the parent compound, has recently received attention as a potentially effective oral agent for the management of enteric fever [522,524–526]. The major advantage of this drug is its increased absorption from the intestine, high blood levels and possibly fewer gastrointestinal side effects. Its bacterial spectrum is identical to that of ampicillin. Cross-resistance between antibiotics is complete. Presently available data indicate that when the same quantities of amoxicillin and ampicillin are administered orally, the former is more effective therapeutically. Oral doses of amoxicillin produce the same results as 100 mg/kg/day of ampicillin given intravenously, but are not as successful as conventional doses of chloramphenicol. Comparison of the efficacy of amoxicillin and trimethoprim-sulfamethoxazole in cases of typhoid fever due to chloramphenicol-resistant or -sensitive organisms has demonstrated that both agents are equally active against the resistant strains, but that trimethoprimsulfamethoxazole is more effective against the sensitive ones. The reason for this lies in the fact that the chloramphenicol-resistant strains failed to be inhibited, while the antibiotic-sensitive ones were suppressed by sulfamethoxazole, thus providing the opportunity for additive or synergistic therapy [526]. Amoxicillin should probably be considered, at this time, as the preferred agent for use in patients who would have been treated orally with ampicillin in the past. The recommended dose of amoxicillin is 4–6 gm, in 4 divided doses per day, for 14 days.

The efficacy of the combination of trimethoprim-sulfamethoxazole (TSM) in the treatment of enteric fevers has been the subject of extensive study [526–540]. Although an occasional nutritionally-depleted individual may manifest evidence of hematologic abnormalities secondary to impairment of the metabolism of folic acid, this preparation appears to be relatively safe. Hematopoietic disorders, when induced, are readily corrected by the administration of folic or folinic acid. In this respect, TSM has considerable advantage over chloramphenicol. It has been demonstrated that 80 to 90% of patients with enteric fever treated with this combination of drugs recover, and do at least as well as those treated with chloramphenicol orally. However, several large studies have indicated that a small number of cases may fail to respond to trimethoprim-sulfamethoxazole therapy, and a few may terminate fatally [533,537,564,565]. The development of resistance of salmonella to the drug has been noted to occur during treatment. It is presently recommended that this combination of antibacterial agents not be used for seriously ill individuals, but be reserved as an alternative for chloramphenicol, especially when the bacteria are resistant to this antibiotic. The dose of trimethoprim-sulfamethoxazole, 80 and 400 mg respectively in each tablet, is 4 to 8 tablets 2 to 3 times per day for 14 days.

As pointed out earlier (Chapter IV), the two most common serious complications of the enteric fevers are ileal perforation and hemorrhage. Because of very poor mobilization of the mesentery and containment of intestinal contents, diffuse peritonitis is almost always the rule when the intestine perforates. Although the salmonella within Peyer's patches and regional lymphoid tissue are responsible for the swelling, ulceration and capillary thrombosis that lead to rupture of the bowel, the organisms that gain entrance to the peritoneal cavity are primarily members of the indigenous intestinal microflora. For this reason, chemotherapy must be directed against the anaerobes and facultative aerobes that constitute this population, as well as against salmonella. The drugs selected for this purpose by different clinicians have varied. We prefer to administer full doses of erythromycin and chloramphenicol. The role of surgical intervention in patients with perforation of the ileum in the course of enteric fever has been controversial. Huckstep [63] and Woodward [513] during the 1960's strongly opposed it, and favored medical management. More recently, however, because of major advances in anesthesiology, control of balance of fluid and electrolytes, the availability of highly effective antimicrobial agents and greater surgical expertise in developing areas of the world where enteric fever is endemic, surgical treatment has been carried out frequently and been noted to produce a significant increase in the rate of survival [286–289,566–568]. Despite the initial impression that surgery would not be successful because the marked thinning of the ileal wall at the site of the perforation might make it difficult for sutures to remain in place, experience has proved this not to be the case. The preferred surgical procedure is wedge resection of the involved area of intestine, if less than 3 holes are present; removal of larger portions of the bowel is reserved for more extensive involvement, or cases in which the bowel is very friable [286,287,566].

The treatment of ileal hemorrhage has traditionally been supportive, and has consisted of transfusions of blood, correction of abnormalities of clotting, if present, etc. This complication of enteric fever may also indicate surgical intervention. Another approach to the management of intestinal bleeding in this disease is illustrated by a case of typhoid fever in which the site of hemorrhage was defined by angiography and then followed by the selective infusion of vasopressin into the involved artery [569]. This resulted in prompt cessation of the hemorrhage, and the patient recovered. More experience with this technic and with the arterial embolization of Gelfoam® into the bleeding vessel is required to establish the effectiveness of these methods as the first steps in the management of intestinal bleeding that may complicate enteric fever.

"SALMONELLA BACTEREMIA"

The primary approach to the management of "*salmonella bacteremia*" and the metastatic infections associated with this syndrome is determination of the level of bacteremia and identification of the sites in which the organisms have focalized. Although bacteria are present continuously in the blood of patients with typhoid and paratyphoid fever, and "salmonella bacteremia," this is quite uncommon with all other syndromes of salmonellosis. The clinical picture of "salmonella bacteremia"—fever, chills, continuous bacteremia due most often to *S. choleraesuis* or *S. typhimurium*—often requires both medical therapy and surgical intervention if a satisfactory rate of survival is to be achieved [331–381]. The first therapy for "salmonella bacteremia" is initiation of chloramphenicol or, if the responsible organism is resistant to this agent, ampicillin if this is proved to be active *in vitro*. Oral treatment should be avoided. An optimal dose of ampicillin is 8 to 12 gm, and of chloramphenicol 4 to 6 gm/day; both should be administered intravenously. Whether or not the combination of trimethoprim and sulfamethoxazole given by mouth is sufficiently effective in this form of disease has not been firmly established. When this preparation is used, 8 to 16 tablets are given in 2 or 3 divided doses per day.

Once antimicrobial therapy has been instituted, a continuous search should be undertaken to detect and identify any site of metastatic spread of the disease. The primary areas of localization of *S. choleraesuis* are the meninges, cardiovascular system, bones and joints. While involvent of the other sites may be readily apparent, there may be some difficulty in localizing infected foci in the heart and blood vessels. Cardiac auscultation, echocardiography, electrocardiography, phonocardiography, cardiac catheterization and cardiac scanning may be of help in identifying lesions in the heart. A search for intravascular involvement, especially the aorto-iliac system, is mandatory. Radionuclide angiography and ultrasound may yield important information [570]. In patients older than 45 years with persistent bacteremia (with *S. choleraesuis, S. typhimurium,* or other serotypes occasionally), particularly those who have had previous vascular surgery or grafts, a search for aneurysms along the course of the aorta and its branches must be carried out. Angiography is very effective in the detection of such lesions. Such aneurysms are usually atherosclerotic, not mycotic, in origin.

Demonstration of the presence of salmonella in the bloodstream of patients with any type of infection produced by this group of organisms mandates intravenous therapy with an effective antimicrobial agent. Although metastatic foci are uncommon in the course of gastroenteritis and enteric fever, the possibility that such a lesion is present must always be considered, especially when treatment does not lead to defervescence, or when manifestations of dysfunction of organs other than those involved in the primary process develop.

Successful management is often difficult in patients with "salmonella bacteremia." This syndrome occurs primarily in patients with underlying disorders, the primary feature of which is episodic acute hemolysis, and in individuals over 50 years of age, who frequently have atherosclerotic aneurysms of the aorta and its main branches. Metastatic focalization of organisms is relatively more common in patients with this type of salmonellosis. For these reasons, it is imperative, especially when relapse occurs within a short time of discontinuation of chemotherapy, that all available technics including arteriography, radionuclide scanning and ultrasound be employed to locate lesions that may be present in the myocardium or on cardiac valves. Demonstration of a single myocardial abscess or endocarditis usually requires surgical intervention while an effective antibacterial drug is being administered. Valvular replacement has been carried out successfully in such cases. Demonstration of an atherosclerotic aneurysm demands removal of the lesion and its replacement with a graft. Our experience suggests that, unless this is done, the clinical course is featured by repeated remissions when an appropriate antibiotic is given, and relapse when it is stopped. Death is the usual outcome when antibacterial agents alone are used. However, when aneurysmectomy is combined with appropriate chemotherapy, the survival rate is strikingly improved. Meade and Moran were the first to report cure of a patient with an aortic aneurysm and bacteremia with *S. typhimurium* by combining medical and surgical therapy [349]. A dacron graft was placed between the site in the aorta where the lesion was removed and the iliac arteries. This procedure may be associated with an appreciable risk of infection of the graft leading to dehiscence of recurrent bacteremia. Because of this, it has been suggested that arterial bypass reconstruction through sterile tissues is the preferred approach. This has been accomplished by careful reconstruction of the peritoneum posterior to the graft, resulting in separation of the prosthesis from the potentially-infected retroperitoneal bed. Perhaps the best way of accomplishing this is by the construction of either a thoraco-iliac or axillo-femoral graft that avoids the infected area completely. Treatment with an effective antibacterial agent by the intravenous route is carried out for 5 to 7 days prior to, during and for 4–6 weeks after operation [335,350,352,353].

The management of extraintestinal, nonvascular metastatic infections caused by salmonella is the same as that employed in the treatment of localized disease due to other bacteria in similar anatomic sites. This includes surgical drainage of the lesion and 10 to 14 days of appropriate antimicrobial therapy. There are, however, a few special situations that may alter this approach. Invasion of bone by salmonella often produces a chronic rather than an acute process. While combined surgery and medical therapy is often required when the osteomyelitis is chronic, the acute infection can usually be eradicated by the intravenous administration of 4 gm of chloramphenicol or an appropriate dose of another active agent for 4 weeks. Meningitis, pneumonia and suppurative arthritis due to this group of organisms are usually controlled with antibiotics alone. Technetium and gallium scanning may be very helpful in identifying the metastatic focus. Infection of the genitourinary tract responds quite favorably to the use of the combination of trimethoprim and sulfamethoxazole, especially in males. High concentrations of both drugs are achieved in the urine and of trimethoprim in prostatic secretions. If necessary, treatment with this agent may be continued for a long period.

THE CARRIER STATE

Gastroenteritis due to salmonella may be followed by either transient (up to 1 year) or permanent (beyond one year) carriage of the organisms in a variable but relatively small number of cases. In most instances, the organisms disappear from the feces in 3 months or less. Carriage is usually limited to the intestine in these patients; persistence of the bacteria in the gallbladder is quite uncommon. Unless there are strong indications that short-term carriers (up to 3 months) constitute a menace to the public health, chemotherapy for eradication of the salmonella is not recommended. In the permanent carriers, the therapy of choice is ampicillin or amoxicillin for 4 weeks. This is followed by culture of stool once weekly for 3 weeks; if still positive, a second course of antibiotic is undertaken.

Patients who have had typhoid or paratyphoid fever are prone to becoming carriers of the *S. typhi* or the paratyphoid organisms in their gallbladder and/

or intrahepatic biliary tree; this is quite uncommon in those who have experienced an episode of acute gastroenteritis caused by other salmonella, and have not developed metastatic infection of or direct spread to the biliary tree. Eradication of the carrier state when the gallbladder is involved poses a difficult problem, even when appropriate doses of chloramphenicol are administered [449,571,572]. Cholecystectomy, without concomitant antimicrobial therapy, results in cure in 70 to 80% of cases, but is associated with a significant morbidity and mortality because of dissemination of the organisms at the time of surgery [571–573]. The administration of 2 to 4 gm of ampicillin orally for 4 weeks has been found effective in eliminating the excretion of organisms in the stool, when gallstones have not been present, in about 80% of patients [574–581]. Studies over 4 to 9 years of the individuals in this group from whom the salmonella have been eliminated suggest that, if relapse does not develop within two years, cure is probably permanent [582]. When cholelithiasis is present, the possibility of eradication of the carrier state is relatively poor [449,451,577]. This is probably related to the fact that, in the presence of chronic cholecystitis, especially if there is any degree of obstruction, most antibiotics fail to get into bile. Also, the stones may serve as a foreign body nidus for the maintenance of continued infection. Treatment with ampicillin combined with cholecystectomy is probably the optimal approach to the solution of this problem; cure is accomplished in over 90% of cases by this combination [451,580]. It has recently been suggested that intravenous administration of ampicillin (8 to 10 gm/day) may be of value in eradication of the carrier state in instances in which relapse has occurred after the drug has been given orally, or in those in whom removal of gallstones is, for some reason, contraindicated [448,583]. Oral therapy with amoxicillin, with or without concomitant probenecid, may be more effective than oral ampicillin, particularly in patients with disease of the biliary tract, because of the greater degree of absorption of the former from the gastrointestinal tract [523]. Preliminary studies of trimethoprim plus sulfamethoxazole have suggested that the effect of this preparation is comparable to that of ampicillin in chronic carriers, and is especially useful in patients sensitized to penicillins, or harboring organisms resistant to ampicillin [584–587]. The present practice of the writers in chronic carriers of salmonella is to administer 1 gm of ampicillin orally every 6 hours for 4 to 6 weeks; if this fails, cholecystectomy is carried out while chemotherapy is being given. Patients who are poor surgical risks or refuse operation, are given 6 to 10 gm of ampicillin per day intravenously, or are treated with amoxicillin; failure with this approach suggests the use of trimethoprim plus sulfamethoxazole.

In the absence of obstructive lesions in the urinary tract, the management of carriage of salmonella in this area involves the same approach as that employed to eradicate the intestinal carrier state in patients free of disease of the biliary tract. Treatment with ampicillin, amoxicillin or trimethoprim-sulfamethoxazole for 4 to 6 weeks is effective. In cases in which obstructing lesions are present, therapy includes surgical correction of the anatomic abnormalities together with administration of an appropriate antimicrobial agent. Effective cure of patients with schistosomiasis of carriage of salmonella in the urine and/or blood necessitates a combined attack on both the parasite and thc bacterium.

Bibliography

1. Edwards PR, Ewing WH: *Identification of Enterobacteriaceae,* Second Edition, Burgess Publishing Co., Minneapolis, 1962, 258 pp.
2. Committee on Salmonella, Division of Biology and Agriculture of the National Research Council: *An Evaluation of the Salmonella Problem.* National Academy of Sciency, Washington, D.C., 1969, 207 pp.
3. Huber TW, Macias EG, Holmes P, Bredthauer HD: A clinical isolate of *Salmonella typhi* requiring anaerobic conditions for primary isolation. Am J Clin Path *63:* 117–119, 1975.
4. Bailey WR, Scott EG: *Diagnostic Microbiology.* Fourth Edition. CV Mosby Co., St. Louis, 1974, 414 pp.
5. Ewing WH, Martin WJ: Enterobacteriaceae, in Lennette EH, Spaulding EH, Truant JP: *Manual of Clinical Microbiology.* Second Edition, American Society for Microbiology, Washington, D.C. 1974, pp. 189–221.
6. Bowmer EJ: The challenge of salmonellosis; major public health problem. Am J Med Sci *247:* 467–501, 1964.
7. Salmonella Subcommittee of Nomenclature Committee of International Society for Microbiology. J Hygiene *34:* 333–350, 1934.
8. Sonnenwirth AC: The enteric bacilli and similar gram-negative bacteria, in Davis BD, Dulbecco R, Eisen HN, Ginsberg HS, Wood WB Jr, McCarty M: *Microbiology,* Second Edition. Harper and Row, New York, 1973, pp. 753–789.
9. Widal F: Serodiagnostic de la fievre typhoide apropos d'une modification par MMC Nicolle et A. Halipue. Bull Soc Med Hosp *13:* 561–566, 1896.
10. Gotoff SP, Lepper MH, Fiedler MA: Immunologic studies in an epidemic of salmonella infections. Am J Med Sci *251:* 22–28, 1966.
11. Diaz F, Neter E: Antibody response to the common enterobacterial antigen of children with shigellosis, salmonellosis or urinary tract infection. Am J Med Sci *256:* 18–24, 1968.
12. Schroeder SA: Interpretation of serologic tests for typhoid fever. JAMA *206:* 839–840, 1968.
13. Stuart BM, Pullen RL: Typhoid; clinical analysis of 360 cases. Arch Int Med *78:* 629–661, 1946.
14. Benenson AS: Serological responses of man to typhoid vaccines. Bull WHO *30:* 653–662, 1964.
15. Vogelsang TM, Wetteland P, Wormnes A: Intradermal versus subcutaneous immunization with typhoid-paratyphoid A and B vaccines in human adults. Acta Path Microbiol Scand *61:* 109–116, 1964.
16. Reynolds DW, Carpenter L, Simon WH: Diagnostic specificity of Widal's reaction for typhoid fever. JAMA *214:* 2192–2193, 1970.
17. Sansone P, Saslaw MS, Hennekens CH Jr: High titer Widal reaction. JAMA *220:* 1615–1616, 1972.

18. Protell RL, Soloway RD, Martin WJ, Schoenfield LJ, Summerskill WHJ: Anti-salmonella agglutinins in chronic active liver disease. Lancet *2:* 330–332, 1971.
19. Nakano M, Saito K: Chemical components in the cell wall of *Salmonella typhimurium* affecting its virulence and immunogenicity in mice. Nature *222:* 1085–1086, 1969.
20. Valtonen V: Virulence of salmonella strains with a reduced amount of 0-antigen. J Gen Microbiol *57:* 28–29, 1969.
21. Mäkelä PH, Valtonen VV, Valtman M: Role of 0-antigen (Lipopolysaccharide) factors in the virulence of *Salmonella.* J Inf Dis *128 Suppl:* 581–585, 1973.
22. Felix A, Pitt RM: The pathogenic and immunogenic activities of *Salmonella typhi* in relation to its antigenic constituents. J Hyg *49:* 92–110, 1915.
23. Hornick RB, Greisman SE, Wodward TE, DuPont HL, Dawkins AT, Snyder MJ: Typhoid fever: pathogenesis and immunologic control. New Engl J Med *283:* 686–691, 739–746, 1970.
24. Hook EW, Johnson WD: Typhoid fever and nontyphoidal salmonellosis in Hoeprich, PD, Ed. *Infectious Diseases.* Harper and Row, Hagerstown, Md., 1972, pp. 583–601.
25. Public Health Laboratory Service Working Party: The detection of the typhoid carrier state. J Hyg *59:*231–247, 1961.
26. Bokkenheuser V, Smit P, Richardson N: A challenge to the validity of the Vi test for the detection of chronic typhoid carriers. Am J Public Health *54:* 1507–1513, 1964.
27. McCabe WR: Immunoprophylaxis of gram-negative bacillary infections. In Creger WP, Coggins CH, Hancock EW, Ed. *Annual Review of Medicine 27:* 335–341, 1976.
28. Wilson GS, Miles A: *Topley and Wilson's Principles of Bacteriology, Virology, and Immunity.* Sixth Edition. Williams and Wilkins, Baltimore, 1975, pp. 358–364, 1282–1290.
29. Elin RJ, Wolff SM: Biology of endotoxin. In Creger WP, Coggins CH, Hancock EW, Ed. *Annual Review of Medicine 27:* 127–141, 1976.
30. Datta N: Epidemiology and classification of plasmids. In Schlessinger D, Ed. *Microbiology-1974.* American Society for Microbiology, Washington, D.C., 1975, pp. 9–15.
31. Novick RP, Clowes RC, Cohen SN, Curtiss R III, Datta N, Falkow S: Uniform nomenclature for bacterial plasmids: a proposal. Bact Rev *40:* 168–189, 1976.
32. McHugh GL, Moellering RC, Hopkins, CC, Swartz MN: *Salmonella typhimurium* resistant to silver nitrate, chloramphenicol, and ampicillin. A new threat in burn units? Lancet *1:* 235–240, 1975.
33. Gangarosa EJ, Bennett JV, Wyatt C, Pierce PE, Olante J, Hernandes PM, Vazquez V, Bessudo DM: An epidemic-associated episome? J Inf Dis *126:* 215–218, 1972.
34. Overturf G, Marton KI, Mathies AW Jr: Antibiotic resistance in typhoid fever; chloramphenicol resistance among clinical isolates of *Salmonella typhosa* in Los Angeles, 1972—Epidemiologic and bacteriologic characteristics. New Engl J Med *289:* 463–465, 1973.
35. Butler T, Linh NN, Arnold K, Pollack M: Chloramphenicol-resistant typhoid fever in Vietnam associated with R factors. Lancet *2:* 983–985, 1975.
36. Anderson ES: The problem and implications of chloramphenicol resistance in the typhoid bacillus. J Hyg *74:* 289–299, 1975.
37. Cohen SN: Chloramphenicol-ampicillin resistant *Salmonella typhi*—California. Morbid Mortal Week Rep *22:* 183, 1973.
38. Olarte J, Galindo E: *Salmonella typhi* resistant to chloramphenicol, ampicillin and other antimicrobial agents: strains isolated during an extensive typhoid fever epidemic in Mexico. Antimicrob Agents Chemother *4:* 596–601, 1973.
39. Olarte J, Galindo E, Joachim A: Sensitivity of salmonella, shigella, and enteropathogenic *Escherichia coli* species to cephalothin, ampicillin, chloramphenicol, and tetracycline. Antimicrobial Agents Chemother *2:* 787–793, 1962.
40. Kaye D, Merselis JG, Hook EW: Susceptibility of salmonella species to four antibiotics. New Engl J Med *269:* 1084–1086, 1963.

41. Smith DH: Salmonella with transferable drug resistance. New Engl J Med *275:* 625–630, 1966.
42. Gill FA, Hook EW: Salmonella strains with transferable antimicrobial resistance. JAMA *198:* 1267–1269, 1966.
43. Schroeder SA, Terry PM, Bennett JV: Antibiotic resistance and transfer factor in salmonella, United States, 1967. JAMA *205:* 903–906, 1968.
44. Adams R, Nelson JD: Susceptibility of salmonellae to cephalosporins and to nine other antimicrobial agents. App Microbiol *16:* 1570–1574, 1968.
45. Manten A, Guinee PAM, Kampelmacher EH, Voogd CE: An eleven year study of drug resistance in salmonella in the Netherlands. Bull WHO *45:* 85–93, 1971.
46. Winshell EB, Cherubin C, Winter J, Neu HC: Antibiotic resistance of salmonella in the eastern United States. *Antimicrobial Agents Chemother 9:* 86–89, 1969.
47. Neu HC, Winshell EB, Winter J, Cherubin CE: Antibiotic resistance of salmonella in northeastern United States 1968–1969. NY State J Med *71:* 1196–1200, 1971.
48. Cherubin CE, Szmuness M, Winter J: Antibiotic resistance of salmonella. NY State J Med *72:* 369–372, 1972.
49. Bissett ML, Abbott SL, Wood PM: Antimicrobial resistance and R factors in *Salmonella* isolated in California (1971–1972). Antimicrob Agents Chemother *5:* 161–168, 1974.
50. Néu HC, Cherubin CE, Longo ED, Flouton B, Winter J: Antimicrobial resistance and R-factor transfer among isolates of *Salmonella* in the Northeastern United States: A comparison of human and animal isolates. J Inf Dis *132:* 617–622, 1975.
51. Pocurull DW, Gaines SA, Mercer HD: Survey of infectious multiple drug resistance among salmonella isolated from animals in the United States. App Microbiol *21:* 358–362, 1971.
52. Anderson ES: Drug resistance in *Salmonella typhimurium* and its implications. Brit Med J *3:* 333–339, 1968.
53. Watanabe T, Arai T, Hattori T: Effects of cell wall polysaccharide on the mating ability of *Salmonella typhimurium.* Nature *225:* 70–71, 1970.
54. Watanabe T: Infectious drug resistance in bacteria. *In Current Topics in Microbiology and Immunology,* no. 56, Springer-Verlag, New York, 1971, pp. 43–98.
55. Aserkoff B, Schroeder SA, Brachman PS: Salmonellosis in the United States—a five-year review. Am J Epidem *92:* 13–24, 1970.
56. Center for Disease Control: Salmonella Surveillance Reports, Annual Summaries 1963–1974.
57. Sanders E, Brachman PS, Friedman EA, Goldsby J, McCall CE: Salmonellosis in the United States; results of nationwide surveillance. Am J Epidem *81:* 370–384, 1965.
58. Cherubin CE, Fodor T, Denmark L, Master C, Fuerst HT, Winter J: The epidemiology of salmonellosis in New York City. Am J Epidem *90:* 112–125, 1969.
59. Gangarosa EJ, Barker WH Jr, Baine WB, Morris GK, Rice PA: Man vs. animal feeds as the source of human salmonellosis. Lancet *1:* 878–879, 1973.
60. Rosenstein BJ: Salmonellosis in infants and children; epidemiologic and therapeutic considerations. J Pediatrics *70:* 1–7, 1967.
61. Rubenstein AD, Feemster RF, Smith HM: Salmonellosis as a public health problem in war-time. Am J Public Health *34:* 841–853, 1944.
62. Leading Article: Typhoid carriers. Brit Med J *1:* 1521–1522, 1964.
63. *Huckstep RL: Typhoid Fever and Other Salmonella Infections.* E and S Livingstone Ltd., Edinburgh, 1962 334 pp.
64. Lumsden LL: An outbreak of typhoid fever caused by milk-borne infection. Public Health Rep *40:* 1302–1315, 1925.
65. Rich ED: A typhoid epidemic traced to cheese. Am J Public Health *13:* 210–215, 1923.
66. Sawyer WA: Ninety-three persons infected by a typhoid carrier at a public dinner. JAMA *63:* 1537–1542, 1914.

67. Scottish Home and Health Department. Departmental Committee of Enquiry. The Aberdeen typhoid outbreak, 1964. Edinburgh, 1964.
68. Leading Article: Aberdeen typhoid outbreak of 1964. Brit Med J *2:* 601–602, 1966.
69. Ash I, McKendrick GDW, Robertson MH, Hughes HL: Outbreak of typhoid fever connected with corned beef. Brit Med J *1:* 1474–1478, 1964.
70. Couper WRM, Newell KW, Payne DJH: An outbreak of typhoid fever associated with canned ox-tongue. Lancet *1:* 1057–1059, 1956.
71. Anderson ES, Hobbs BC: Studies of the strain of *Salmonella typhi* responsible for the Aberdeen typhoid outbreak. Isreal J Med Sci *9:* 162–174, 1973.
72. Leading Article: Aberdeen's typhoid bacillus. Lancet *1:* 645–646, 1973.
73. Feldman RE, Baine WB, Nitzkin JL, Saslaw MS, Pollard RA Jr: Epidemiology of *Salmonella typhi* infection in a migrant labor camp in Dade County, Florida. J Inf Dis *130:* 334–342, 1974.
74. Gonzalez-Cortes A, Bessudo D, Sanchez-Leyva R, Fragoso R, Hinojosa M, Becerril P: Water-borne transmission of chloramphenicol-resistant *Salmonella typhi* in Mexico. Lancet *2:* 605–607, 1973.
75. Waldvogel FA, Pitton JS: Typhoid fever imported from Mexico to Switzerland. Studies on R factor mediated chloramphenicol resistance. J Hyg *71:* 509–513, 1973.
76. Anderson ES, Smith HR: Chloramphenicol resistance in the typhoid bacillus. Brit Med J *3:* 329–331, 1972.
77. Lawrence RM, Goldstein E, Hoeprich PD: Typhoid fever caused by chloramphenicol-resistant organisms. JAMA *224:* 861–863, 1973.
78. Bennett IL Jr, Hook EW: Some aspects of salmonellosis. In Rytand DA, Ed. Annual Review of Medicine *10:* 1–20, 1959.
79. Leading Article: Salmonellosis in meat. Brit Med J *2:* 1281, 1964.
80. Atkinson N, Woodroofe GM, Culver DE: Occurrence of salmonella types in Australia. Austral J Exp Biol Med Sci *30:* 73–80, 1952.
81. George JTA, Wallace JG, Morrison HR, Harbourne JF: Paratyphoid in man and cattle. Brit Med J *3:* 208–211, 1972.
82. Eickhoff TC: Salmonellae on the grocery shelf. Ann Int Med *66:* 1279–1283, 1967.
83. McCoy JH: Trends in salmonella food poisoning in England and Wales 1941–1972. J Hyg *74:* 271–282, 1975.
84. Perelli-Minetti JE, Rucker JC, Ross FK: Paratyphoid. Calif Dept Agric Bull *37:* 151–156, 1948.
85. Wilder AN, MacCready RA: Isolation of salmonella from poultry: poultry products and poultry processing plants in Massachusetts. New Engl J Med *274:* 1453–1460, 1966.
86. Ager EA, Nelson KE, Galton MM, Boring JR, Jernigan JR: Two outbreaks of egg-borne salmonellosis and implications for their prevention. JAMA *199:* 372–378, 1967.
87. Collins RS, Treger MD, Goldsby JB, Boring JR, Coohon DB, Barr RN: Salmonella infections traced to powdered milk. JAMA *203:* 838–844, 1968.
88. Galton MM, Lowery WD, Hardy AV: Salmonella in fresh and smoked pork sausage. J Inf Dis *95:* 232–235, 1954.
89. Gangarosa EJ, Bisno AL, Eichner ER, Treger MD, Goldfield M, DeWitt WE, Fodov T, Fish SM, Dougherty WJ, Murphy JB, Feldman J, Vogel H: Epidemic of febrile gastroenteritis due to *Salmonella java* traced to smoked whitefish. Am J Public Health *58:* 114–121, 1968.
90. Craven PC, Mackel DC, Baine WB, Marker WH, Gangarosa EJ, Goldfield M, Rosenfield H, Altman R, Lachapelle G, Davies JW, Swanson RC: International outbreak of *Salmonella eastbourne* infection traced to contaminated chocolate. Lancet *1:* 788–792, 1975.
91. Lee JA: Recent trends in human salmonellosis in England and Wales: the epidemiology of prevalent serotypes other than *Salmonella typhimurium*. J Hyg *72:* 185–195, 1974.
92. Steele JH: Salmonellosis; a major zoonosis. Arch Environ Health *19:*871–875, 1969.

93. Kunz LJ, Ouchterlony OTG: Salmonellosis originating in a hospital: a newly recognized source of infection. New Engl J Med *253:* 761–763, 1955.
94. McCall CE, Collins RS, Jones DB, Kauffman AF, Brachman PS: An interstate outbreak of salmonellosis traced to a contaminated food supplement. Am J Epidem *84:* 32–39, 1966.
95. Lang DJ, Kunz LJ, Martin AR, Schroeder SA, Thomson LA: Carmine as a source of nosocomial salmonellosis. New Engl J Med *276:* 829–832, 1967.
96. Lang DJ, Schroeder SA, Kunz LJ, Thomson LA, Hobbs BC, Butler NJ: Salmonella-contaminated carmine dye. Another example of in-plant contamination during processing. Am J. Public Health *61:* 1615–1619, 1971.
97. Bowmer EJ: Salmonellae: Ubiquitous pathogens of animals and man. Canad J Public Health *59:* 408–410, 1968.
98. Levy BS, McIntire W: The economic impact of a food-borne salmonellosis outbreak. JAMA *230:* 1281–1282, 1974.
99. Brachman PS, Goldsby JB: Salmonella surveillance program in the United States. In *Proceedings of the National Conference on Salmonellosis, 1964.* Public Health Service Publication No. 1262, 1965, pp. 13–17.
100. McCall CE: Identifying outbreaks. *In Proceedings of the National Conference on Salmonellosis, 1964.* Public Health Service Publication No. 1262, 1965, pp. 43–46.
101. Clark GM, Kaufmann AF, Gangarosa EJ, Thompson MA: Epidemiology of an international outbreak of *Salmonella agona.* Lancet *2:* 490–493, 1973.
102. Lamm SH, Taylor A Jr, Gangarosa EJ, Anderson HW, Young W, Clark MH, Bruce AR: Turtle-associated salmonellosis. I. An estimation of the magnitude of the problem in the United States, 1970–1971. Am J Epidem *95:* 511–517, 1972.
103. Schroeder SA, Aserkoff B, Brachman PS: Epidemic salmonellosis in hospitals and institutions; a 5-year review. New Engl J Med *279:* 674–678, 1968.
104. Baine WB, Gangarosa EJ, Bennett JV, Barker WH Jr: Institutional salmonellosis. J Inf Dis *128:* 357–360, 1973.
105. Rice PA, Craven PC, Wells JG: *Salmonella heidelberg* enteritis and bacteremia; an epidemic in two pediatric wards. Am J Med *60:* 509–516, 1976.
106. MacGregor RR, Reinhart J: Person-to-person spread of salmonella: a problem in hospitals? Lancet *2:* 1001–1003, 1973.
107. Pether JVS, Gilbert RJ: The survival of salmonella on finger-tips and transfer of the organisms to foods. J Hyg *69:* 673–681, 1971.
108. Steere AC, Craven PJ, Hall WJ III, Leotsakis N, Wells JG, Farmer JJ III, Gangarosa EJ: Person-to-person spread of *Salmonella typhimurium* after a hospital common-source outbreak. Lancet *1:* 319–322, 1975.
109. Sanders E, Sweeney FJ Jr, Friedman EA, Boring JR, Randall EL, Polk LD: An outbreak of hospital-associated infections due to *Salmonella derby.* JAMA *186:* 984–986, 1963.
110. Pearson HE, Grant WJ: Presumed transmission of salmonella by sigmoidoscope. Calif Med *53:* 23–25, 1970.
111. Rhame FS, Root RK, MacLowry JD, Dadisman TH, Bennett JV: Salmonella septicemia from platelet transfusions. Study of an outbreak traced to a hematogenous carrier of *Salmonella choleraesuis.* Ann Int Med *78:* 633–641, 1973.
112. Chmel H, Armstrong D: *Salmonella oslo*: a focal outbreak in a hospital. Am J Med *60:* 203–208, 1976.
113. Newell KW: Possibilities for investigation and control of salmonellosis for this decade. Am J Public Health *57:* 472–476, 1967.
114. McCullough NB, Eisele CW: Experimental human salmonellosis. I. Pathogenicity of strains of *Salmonella meleagridis* and *Salmonella anatum* obtained from spray-dried whole egg. J Inf Dis *88:* 278–289, 1951.
115. McCullough NB, Eisele CW: Experimental human salmonellosis. II. Immunity studies

following experimental illness with *Salmonella meleagridis* and *Salmonella anatum*. J Immun *66*. 595–608, 1951.

116. McCullough NB, Eisele CW: Experimental human salmonellosis. III. Pathogenicity of strains of *Salmonella newport, Salmonella derby,* and *Salmonella bareilly* obtained from spray-dried whole egg. J Inf Dis *89:* 209–213, 1951.
117. McCullough NB, Eisele CW: Experimental human salmonellosis. IV. Pathogenicity of strains of *Salmonella pullorum* obtained from spray-dried whole egg. J Inf Dis *89:* 259–265, 1951.
118. Silverstolpe L, Plazikowski U, Kjellander J, Vahlne G: An epidemic among infants caused by *Salmonella muenchen*. J Appl Bact *24:* 134–142, 1961.
119. Giannella RA, Broitman SA, Zamcheck N: The gastric barrier to microorganisms in man: *in vivo* and *in vitro* studies. Gut *13:* 251–256, 1972.
120. Giannella RA, Broitman SA, Zamcheck N: Influence of gastric acidity on bacterial and parasitic enteric infections; a perspective. Ann Int Med *78:* 271–276, 1973.
121. Franklin MA, Skoryna SC: Studies on natural gastric flora. I. Bacterial flora of fasting human subjects. Canad Med Assoc J *95:* 1349–1355, 1966.
122. Gray JDA, Shiner M: Influence of gastric pH on gastric and jejunal flora. Gut *8:* 574–581, 1967.
123. Draser BS, Shiner M, McLeod GM: Studies on the intestinal flora. I. The bacterial flora of the gastrointestinal tract in healthy and achlorhydric persons. Gastroenterol *56:* 71–79, 1969.
124. DuPont HL, Hornick RB, Snyder MJ, Libonati JP, Woodward TE: Immunity in typhoid fever: evaluation of live streptomycin-dependent vaccine. Antimicrob Agents Chemother *10:* 236–239, 1971.
125. Collins FM: Salmonellosis in orally infected specific pathogen-free C57B1 mice. Infect Immun *5:* 191–198, 1972.
126. Waddell WR, Kunz LJ: Association of salmonella enteritis with operation of the stomach. New Engl J Med *255:* 555–559, 1956.
127. Close AS, Smith MB, Koch ML, Ellison EH: An analysis of ten cases of salmonella infection on a general surgical service. Arch Surg *80:* 972–976, 1960.
128. Sokol EM: *Salmonella derby* infections after gastrointestinal surgery. Mt Sinai J Med NY *32:* 36–41, 1965.
129. Nordbring F: Contraction of salmonella gastroenteritis following previous operation on the stomach. Acta Med Scand *171:* 783–790, 1962.
130. Giannella RA, Broitman SA, Zamcheck N: Salmonella enteritis. I. Role of reduced gastric secretion in pathogenesis. Am J Dig Dis *16:* 1000–1006, 1971.
131. Giannella RA, Broitman SA, Zamcheck N: Salmonella enteritis. II. Fulminant diarrhea in and effects on the small intestine. Am J Dig Dis *16:* 1007–1013, 1971.
132. Gray JA, Trueman AM: Severe salmonella gastroenteritis associated with hypochlorhydria. Scot Med J *16:* 255–258, 1971.
133. A collaborative report: A waterborne epidemic of salmonellosis in Riverside, California, 1965. Am J Epid *93:* 33–48, 1971.
134. Sprinz H, Gangarosa EJ, Williams M, Hornick RB, Woodward TE: Histopathology of the upper small intestines in typhoid fever. Biopsy study of experimental disease in man. Am J Dig Dis *11:* 615–624, 1966.
135. Takeuchi A: Penetration of the intestinal epithelium by various microorganisms. Curr Top Path *54:* 1–27, 1971.
136. Blacklow NR, Dolin R, Fedson DS, DuPont HL, Northrup RS, Hornick RB, Chanock RM: Acute infectious nonbacterial gastroenteritis: etiology and pathogenesis. Ann Int Med *76:* 993–1008, 1972.
137. WHO Scientific Group: Oral Enteric Bacterial Vaccines. *WHO Tech Rep Sci,* 1972, No. 500.

138. Carter PB, Collins FM: The route of enteric infection in normal mice. J Exp Med *139:* 1189–1203, 1974.
139. Takeuchi A: Election microscope studies of experimental salmonella infection. I. Penetration into the intestinal epithelium by *Salmonella typhimurium.* Am J Path *50:* 109–136, 1967.
140. Takeuchi A, Sprinz H: Electron-microscope studies of experimental salmonella infection in the preconditioned guinea pig. II. Response of the intestinal mucosa to the invasion by *Salmonella typhimurium.* Am J Path *51:* 137–161, 1967.
141. Gaines S, Sprinz H, Tully JG, Tigertt WD: Studies on infection and immunity in experimental typhoid fever. VII. The distribution of *Salmonella typhi* in chimpanzee tissue following oral challenge, and the relationship between the numbers of bacilli and morphologic lesions. J Inf Dis *118:* 293–300, 1968.
142. Giannella RA, Formal SB, Dammin GJ, Collins HJ: Pathogenesis of salmonellosis. Studies of fluid secretion, mucosal invasion, and morphologic reaction in the rabbit ileum. J Clin Invest *52:* 441–453, 1973.
143. Kent TH, Formal SB, LaBrec EH: Salmonellae virulence testing. Arch Path *84:* 300–303, 1967.
144. Osler W: *The Principles and Practice of Medicine,* D. Appleton Co, New York, Seventh Edition, 1909, pp. 57–105.
145. Mallory FB: *The Principles of Pathologic Histology,* WB Saunders Company, Philadelphia, 1914, pp. 162–178.
146. Boyd W: *A Textbook of Pathology; Structure and Function in Disease.* Lea and Febiger, Philadelphia, Eighth Edition, 1970, pp. 326–330.
147. Anderson WAD: *Pathology,* CV Mosby Company, St. Louis, Sixth Edition, 1971, pp. 305–308.
148. Robbins SL: *Pathologic Basis of Disease,* WB Saunders, Philadelphia, Third Edition, 1974, pp. 397–400.
149. Sitprija V, Pipatanagul V, Boonpucknavig V, Boonpucknavig S: Glomerulitis in typhoid fever. Ann Int Med *81:* 210–213, 1974.
150. Powell DW, Plotkin GR, Maenza RM, Solberg LI, Catlin OH, Formal SB: Experimental diarrhea: I. Intestinal water and electrolyte transport in rat salmonella enterocolitis. Gastroenterology *60:* 1053–1064, 1971.
151. Powell DW, Plotkin GR, Solberg LI, Catlin OH, Maenza RM, Formal SB: Experimental diarrhea: II. Glucose-stimulated sodium and water transport in rat salmonella enterocolitis. Gastroenterology *60:* 1065–1075, 1971.
152. Powell DW, Solberg LI, Plotkin GR, Catlin OH, Maenza RM, Formal SB: Experimental diarrhea: III. Bicarbonate transport in rat salmonella enterocolitis. Gastroenterology *60:* 1076–1086, 1971.
153. Fromm D, Giannella RA, Formal SB, Quijano R, Collins H: Ion transport across isolated ileal mucosa invaded by salmonella. Gastroenterol *66:* 215–225, 1974.
154. Giannella RA, Rout WR, Formal SB, Collins H: Role of plasma filtration in the intestinal fluid secretion mediated by infection with *Salmonella typhimurium.* Infect Immun *13:* 470–474, 1976.
155. Rout WR, Formal SB, Dammin GJ, Giannella RA: Pathophysiology of salmonella diarrhea in the Rhesus monkey: intestinal transport, morphological and bacteriological studies. Gastroenterol *67:* 59–70, 1974.
156. Field M: Ion transport in rabbit ileal mucosa. II. Effects of cyclic 3′,5′-AMP. Am J Physiol *221:* 992–997, 1971.
157. Field M, Fromm D, Al-Awqati Q, Greenough WB III: Effect of cholera enterotoxin on ion transport across isolated ileal mucosa. J Clin Invest *51:* 796–804, 1972.
158. Gots RE, Formal SB, Giannella RA: Salmonella-mediated ileal secretion: stimulation of adenyl cyclase, inhibition by indomethacin and possible participation of prostaglandins. Clin Res *22:* 358A, 1974.

159. Giannella RA, Gots RE, Charney AN, Greenough WB III, Formal SB: Pathogenesis of salmonella-mediated intestinal fluid secretion: Activation of adenylate cyclase and inhibition by indomethacin. Gastroenterol *69:* 1238–1245, 1975.
160. Sharp GWG, Hynie S: Stimulation of intestinal adenyl cyclase by cholera toxin. Nature *229:* 266–269, 1971.
161. Kimberg DV, Field M, Johnson J, Henderson A, Gershon E: Stimulation of intestinal mucosal adenyl cyclase by cholera enterotoxin and prostaglandins. J Clin Invest *50:* 1218–1230, 1971.
162. Harris JC, DuPont HL, Hornick RB: Fecal leukocytes in diarrheal illness. Ann Int Med *76:* 697–703, 1972.
163. Sprinz H: Pathogenesis of intestinal infections. Arch Path *87:* 556–562, 1969.
164. Masson PL, Heremans JF, Schonne E: Lactoferrin, an iron-binding protein in neutrophilic leukocytes. J Exp Med *130:* 643–658, 1969.
165. Faulk WP, Rider JA, Swader JI: Proteins in gastric juice: a study of fifty cases. J Lab Clin Med *77:* 228–238, 1971.
166. Gotze O, Muller-Eberhard H: The C3-activator system: an alternate pathway of complement activation. J Exp Med *134* (Suppl): 90S-108S, 1971.
167. Baggs RB, Miller SA: Nutritional iron deficiency as a determinant of host resistance in the rat. J Nutrition *103:* 1554–1560, 1973.
168. Baggs RB, Miller SA: Defect in resistance to *Salmonella typhimurium* in iron-deficient rats. J Inf Dis *130:* 409–411, 1974.
169. Nissle A: Ueber die Grundlagen einer ursaechlichen Bekaempfung der pathologischen Darmflora. Deut Med Worchosch *42:* 1181–1184, 1916.
170. Bohnhoff M, Drake BL, Miller CP: Effect of streptomycin on susceptibility of intestinal tract to salmonella infection. Proc Soc Expt Biol Med *86:* 133–137, 1954.
171. Miller CP, Bohnhoff M: Changes in the mouse's enteric microflora associated with enhanced susceptibility to salmonella infection following streptomycin treatment. J Inf Dis *113:* 59–66, 1963.
172. Meynell GG: Antibacterial mechanisms of the mouse gut. II. The role of E_h and volatile fatty acids in the normal gut. Brit J Exp Path *44:* 209–219, 1963.
173. Bohnhoff M, Miller CP, Martin WR: Resistance of the mouse's intestinal tract to experimental salmonella infection. I. Factors which interfere with the initiation of infection by oral inoculation. J Exp Med *120:* 805–816, 1964.
174. Bohnhoff M, Miller CP, Martin WR: Resistance of the mouse's intestinal tract to experimental salmonella infection. II. Factors responsible for its loss following streptomycin treatment. J Exp Med *120:* 817–828, 1964.
175. Hentges DJ: Enteric pathogen—normal flora interactions. Am J Clin Nutrit *23:* 1451–1456, 1970.
176. Wawszkiewicz EJ, Schneider HA, Starcher B, Pollack J, Nielands JB: Salmonellosis pacifarin activity of enterobacteria. Proc Nat Acad Sci *68:* 2870–2873, 1971.
177. Collins FM: Immunity to enteric infection in mice. Infect Immun *1:* 243–250, 1970.
178. Cooper GN, Fahey KJ: Oral immunization in experimental salmonellosis. III. Behavior of virulent and temperature-sensitive mutant strains in the intestinal tissues of rats. Infect Immun *2:* 192–200, 1970.
179. Hsu HS, Radcliffe AS: Interactions between macrophages of guinea pigs and salmonellae. J Bact *96:* 191–197, 1968.
180. Mitsuhashi S, Sata I, Tanaka T: Experimental salmonellosis: intracellular growth of *Salmonella enteritidis* ingested in mononuclear phagocytes of mice and cellular basis of immunity. J Bact *81:* 863–868, 1961.
181. Blanden RV, MacKaness GB, Collins FM: Mechanisms of acquired resistance in mouse typhoid. J Exp Med *124:* 585–600, 1966.

182. MacKaness GB, Blanden RV, Collins FM: Mechanisms of acquired resistance in mouse typhoid. J Exp Med *124:* 573–583, 1966.
183. Wagner HN Jr, Elio M, Hornick RB: Studies of the reticuloendothelial system (RES). II. Changes in the phagocytic capacity of the RES in patients with certain infections. J Clin Invest *42:* 427–434, 1963.
184. Greisman SE, Wagner HN Jr, Ilio M, Hornick RB: Mechanisms of endotoxin tolerance. II. Relationship between endotoxin tolerance and reticuloendothelial system phagocytic activity in man. J Exp Med *119:* 241–264, 1964.
185. Hopps HE, Smadel JE, Bernheim BC, Danauskas JX, Jackson EB: Effect of antibiotics on intracellular *Salmonella typhosa.* II. Elimination of infection by prolonged treatment. J Immun *87:* 162–174, 1961.
186. Hornick RB, Woodward TE, McCrumb FR, Snyder MJ, Dawkins AT, Bulkeley JT, De La Macourra F, Corizza FA: Typhoid fever vaccine—yes or no? Med Clin North Amer *51:* 617–623, 1967.
187. Hornick RB, Woodward TE: Appraisal of typhoid vaccine in experimentally infected human subjects. Trans Amer Clin Climat Assoc *78:* 70–78, 1967.
188. Miller RM, Garbus J, Hornick RB: Lack of enhanced oxygen consumption by polymorphonuclear leukocytes on phagocytosis of virulent *Salmonella typhi.* Science *175:* 1010–1011, 1972.
189. Dimitrov NV, Douwes F: Metabolic deficiency of polymorphonuclear leukocytes in sickle-cell disease. J Clin Invest *49:* 82a, 1970.
190. Moellering RC Jr, Weinberg AN: Persistent salmonella infection in a female carrier for chronic granulomatous disease. Ann Int Med *73:* 595–601, 1970.
191. Cherubin CE, Neu HC, Imperato PJ, Harvey RP, Bellen N: Septicemia with non-typhoid salmonella. Medicine *53:* 365–376, 1974.
192. Webster LT: Inheritance and acquired factors in resistance to infection. I. Development of resistant and susceptible lines of mice through selective breeding. J Exp Med *57:* 793–817, 1933.
193. Gowen JW: Genetic effects in nonspecific resistance to infectious disease. Bacteriol Rev *24:* 192–200, 1960.
194. Plant J, Glynn AA: Natural resistance to *Salmonella* infection, delayed hypersensitivity and Ir genes in different strains of mice. Nature *248:* 345–347, 1974.
195. Plant J, Glynn AA: Genetics of resistance to infection with *Salmonella typhimurium* in mice. J Inf Dis *133:* 72–78, 1976.
196. MacKaness GB: Resistance to intracellular infection. J Inf Dis, *123:* 439–445, 1971.
197. Allardyce RA, Shearman DJC, McClelland DBL, Marwick K, Simpson AJ, Laidlaw RB: Appearance of specific colostrum antibodies after clinical infection with *Salmonella typhimurium.* Brit Med J *3:* 307–309, 1974.
198. Marmion DE, Naylor GRE, Stewart IO: Second attacks of typhoid fever. J Hygiene *51:* 260–267, 1953.
199. Cvjetanovic B, Vemura K: The present status of field and laboratory studies of typhoid and paratyphoid vaccines. Bull WHO *32:* 29–36, 1965.
200. Hejfec LB, Salmin LV, Lejtman MZ, Kuz 'minova ML, Vasileva AV, Levina LA, Bencianova TG, Paulova EA, Antonova AA: A controlled field trial and laboratory study of five typhoid vaccines in the USSR. Bull WHO *34:* 321–339, 1966.
201. Watson KC: The relapse state in typhoid fever treated with chloramphenicol. Am J Trop Med Hyg *6:* 72–80, 1957.
202. Spaun J, Vemura K: International reference preparations of typhoid vaccine. Bull WHO *31:* 761–791, 1964.
203. Schubert AF, Hornick RB, Ewald RW: Changes of serum complement and properdin levels in experimental typhoid fever: a longitudinal study of the disease including the incubation

period and the phase of recovery following treatment with chloramphenicol. J Immunol *93:* 387–396, 1964.

204. Kumar R, Maliviga AN, Murthy RGS, Venkataraman M, Mohapatra LN: Immunological study of typhoid: immunoglobulins, C3, antibodies, and leukocyte migration inhibition in patients with typhoid fever and TAB-vaccinated individuals. Infect Immun *10:* 1219–1225, 1974.
205. Douglas SD, Goldberg LS, Fudenberg HH: Clinical, serologic, and leukocyte function studies on patients with idiopathic "acquired" agammaglobulinemia and their families. Am J Med *48:* 48–53, 1970.
206. Stites DP, Levin AS, Lauer BA, Costom BH, Fudenberg HH: Selective "dysgammaglobulinemia" with elevated serum IgA levels and chronic salmonellosis. Am J Med *54:* 260–264, 1973.
207. Dupuis F, Vereerstraeten P, Van Geertruyden J, Kinnaert P, Schoutens E, Toussaint C: *Salmonella typhimurium* infection after kidney transplantation. Report of seven cases. Clin Nephrol *2:* 131–135, 1974.
208. Fiser RH, Denniston JC, Beisel WR: Infection with *Diplococcus pneumoniae* and *Salmonella typhimurium* in monkeys: changes in plasma lipids and lipoproteins. J Inf Dis *125:* 54–60, 1972.
209. Wannemacher RW Jr, DuPont HL, Pekarek RS, Powanda MC, Schwartz A, Hornick RB, Beisel WR: An endogenous mediator of depression of amino acids and trace metals in serum during typhoid fever. J Inf Dis *126:* 77–86, 1972.
210. Pekarek RS, Kluge RM, DuPont HL, Wannemacher RW Jr, Hornick RB, Bostian KA, Beisel WR: Serum zinc, iron, and copper concentrations during typhoid fever in man: effect of chloramphenicol therapy. Clin Chem *21:* 528–532, 1975.
211. Feigen RD, Klainer AS, Beisel WR, Hornick RB: Whole-blood amino acids in experimentally-induced typhoid fever in man. New Engl J Med *278:* 293–298, 1968.
212. Williams G, Newberne PM: Effects of infection on selected clinical and biochemical parameters in dogs. Brit J Exp Path *51:* 253–264, 1970.
213. Lutz JH, Gregerman RI, Spaulding SW, Hornick RB, Dawkins AT Jr: Thyroxine binding proteins, free thyroxine, and thyroxine turnover interrelationships during acute infectious illness in man. J Clin Endocrin Metab *35:* 230–249, 1972.
214. Wolff SM: Biological effects of bacterial endotoxins in man. J Infect Dis *128* (Suppl): 259–264, 1973.
215. Atkins EA, Bodel P: Fever. New Engl J Med *286:* 27–34, 1972.
216. Bennett IL Jr, Petersdorf RG, Keene WR: The pathogenesis of fever: Evidence for direct cerebral action of bacterial endotoxin. Trans Assoc Am Phys *60:* 64–72, 1957.
217. Greisman SE, Hornick RB, Woodward TE: The role of endotoxin during typhoid fever and tularemia in man. III. Hyperreactivity to endotoxin during infection. J Clin Invest *43:* 1747–1757, 1964.
218. Greisman SE, Hornick RB, Carozza FA Jr, Woodward TE: The role of endotoxin during typhoid fever and tularemia in man. I. Acquisition of tolerance to endotoxin. J Clin Invest *42:* 1064–1075, 1963.
219. Horowitz HI, Des Prez RM, Hook EW: Effects of bacterial endotoxin on rabbit platelets. II. Enhancement of platelet factor 3 activity *in vitro* and *in vivo*. J Exp Med *116:* 619–633, 1962.
220. Morrison DC, Cochrane CG: Direct evidence for Hageman factor (factor XII) activation by bacterial lipopolysaccharides (endotoxins). J Exp Med *140:* 797–811, 1974.
221. Mergenhagen SE, Snyderman R, Gewurz H, Shin HS: Significance of complement to the mechanism of action of endotoxin. Curr Top Microbiol Immunol *50:* 37–77, 1969.
222. Frank MM, May JE, Kane MA: Contributions of the classical and alternate complement pathways to the biological effects of endotoxin. J Infec Dis *128* (Suppl): 176–181, 1973.

223. Fine DP: Activation of the classic and alternate complement pathways by endotoxin. J Immunol *112:* 763–769, 1974.
224. Hinshaw LB, Brake CM, Emerson TE Jr: Biochemical and pathologic alterations in endotoxin shock. *In* Mills LJ, Moyer JH (eds.): *Shock and Hypotension: Pathogenesis and Treatment.* Grune and Stratton, New York, 1965, pp. 431–441.
225. Lillehei RC, Longerbeam JK, Bloch JH, Manax WG: Hemodynamic changes in endotoxin shock. *In* Mills LJ, Moyer JH (eds.): *Shock and Hypotension: Pathogenesis and Treatment.* Grune and Stratton, New York, 1965, pp. 442–462.
226. Cho YW: Direct cardiac action of *E. coli* endotoxin. Proc Soc Exp Biol Med *141:* 705–707, 1972.
227. Athens JW, Haab OP, Raab SO, Mauer AM, Ashenbrucker H, Cartwright GE, Wintrobe MM: Leukokinetic studies. IV. The total blood, circulating and marginal granulocyte pools and the granulocyte turnover rate in normal subjects. J Clin Invest *40:* 989–995, 1961.
228. Marsh JC, Perry S: The granulocyte response to endotoxin in patients with hematological disorders. Blood *23:* 581–599, 1964.
229. Sheagren JN, Wolff SM, Shulman NR: Febrile and hematologic responses of rhesus monkeys to bacterial endotoxin. Am J Physiol *212:* 884–890, 1967.
230. McKay DG, Margaretten W, Csavossy I: An electron microscope study of the effects of bacterial endotoxin on the blood-vascular system. Lab Invest *15:* 1815–1829, 1966.
231. Stetson CA Jr: Studies on the mechanisms of the Shwartzman phenomenon. Certain factors involved in the production of the local hemorrhagic necrosis. J Exp Med *93:* 489–504, 1951.
232. Spielvogel AR: An ultrastructural study of the mechanisms of platelet-endotoxin interaction. J Exp Med *126:* 235–250, 1967.
233. Das J, Schwartz AA, Folkman J: Clearance of endotoxin by platelets: Role in increasing the accuracy of the Limulus gelation test and in combating experimental endotoxemia. Surgery *74:* 235–240, 1973.
234. Carroll BJ, Pearson MJ, Martin FIR: Evaluation of three acute tests of hypothalamic-pituitary-adrenal function. Metabolism *18:* 476–483, 1969.
235. Frohman LA, Horton ES, Lebovitz HE: Growth hormone releasing action of a *Pseudomonas* endotoxin (Piromen). Metabolism *16:* 57–67, 1967.
236. Kohler PO, O'Malley BW, Rayford PL, Lipsett MB, Odell WD: Effect of pyrogen on blood levels of pituitary tropic hormones. Observations of the usefulness of the growth hormone response in the detection of pituitary disease. J Clin Endocrinol Metab *27:* 219–226, 1967.
237. Jeffries CD: Liver carbohydrate levels in mice treated with endotoxin, cortisone, and elipten. Proc Soc Exp Biol Med *130:* 413–417, 1969.
238. Shands JW Jr, Miller V, Martin H, Senterfitt V: Hypoglycemic activity of endotoxin. II. Mechanisms of the phenomenon in BCG-infected mice. J Bacteriol *98:* 494–501, 1969.
239. Shtasel TF, Berry LJ: Effect of endotoxin and cortisone on synthesis of ribonucleic acid and protein in livers of mice. J Bacteriol *97:* 1018–1025, 1969.
240. Elin RJ, Wolff SM: Effect of fever on serum iron in man. Clin Res *21:* 598, 1973.
241. Kampschmidt RF, Schultz GA: Hypoferremia in rats following injection of bacterial endotoxin. Proc Soc Exp Biol Med *106:* 870–871, 1961.
242. Kampschmidt RF, Upchurch HF: Effect of endotoxin upon total iron-binding capacity of the serum. Proc Soc Exp Biol Med *116:* 420–422, 1964.
243. Kampschmidt RF, Upchurch HF: A comparison of the effects of rabbit endogenous pyrogen on the body temperature of the rabbit and lowering of plasma iron in the rat. Proc Soc Exp Biol Med *133:* 128–130, 1970.
244. Pekarek RS, Beisel WR: Effect of endotoxin on serum zinc concentrations in the rat. Appl Microbiol *18:* 482–484, 1969.
245. Gery I, Kruger J, Spiesel SZ: Stimulation of B-lymphocytes by endotoxin. J Immunol *108:* 1088–1091, 1972.

246. Peary DL, Shands JW Jr, Adler WH, Smith RT: Mitogenicity of bacterial endotoxins: Characterization of the mitogenic principle. J Immunol *111:* 352–357, 1973.
247. Neter E: Endotoxins and the immune response. Curr Top Microbiol Immunol *47:* 82–124, 1969.
248. McMaster PD, Fanzi RE: The primary immune response in mice. II. Cellular responses of lymphoid tissue accompanying the enhancement or complete suppression of antibody formation by a bacterial endotoxin. J Exp Med *121:* 1109–1125, 1968.
249. Seligmann E, Saphra I, Wasserman M: Salmonella infections in man: analysis of 1000 cases bacteriologically identified by New York Salmonella Center. Am J Hyg *38:* 226–249, 1943.
250. Saphra I, Winter JW: Clinical manifestations of salmonellosis in man: evaluation of 7779 human infections identified at New York Salmonella Center. New Engl J Med *256:* 1128–1134, 1957.
251. Black PH, Kunz LJ, Swartz MN: Salmonellosis—a review of some unusual aspects. New Engl J Med *262:* 811–817, 864–870, 921–927, 1960.
252. Axon ATR, Poole D: Salmonellosis presenting with cholera-like diarrhea. Lancet *1:* 745–746, 1973.
253. Dolman CE, Hudson VG, Malcolm MM, Kerr DE: Salmonella-shigella infections in British Columbia in 1942–52. Canad J Public Health *44:* 27, 1953.
254. Wetherbee DG, Anderson DT, Kuhns DM: Isolation of three Salmonella types from one case of salmonellosis. Texas Rep Biol Med *7:* 397–402, 1949.
255. Hormaeche E, Surraco NL, Pefluffo CA, Aleppo PL: Causes of infantile summer diarrhea. Am J Dis Child *66:* 539–551, 1943.
256. Juenker AP: Infection with multiple types of salmonellae. Am J Clin Path *27:* 646–651, 1957.
257. Faiman J, Rabinowitz JG, Meyers MA: Roentgenology of infectious colitis. Am J Roentgen, Rad Ther, Nucl Med *119:* 375–381, 1973.
258. Kazemi M, Gumpert G, Marks MI: Clinical spectrum and carrier state of nontyphoidal salmonella infections in infants and children. Canad Med Assoc J *110:* 1253–1257, 1974.
259. Stein H, Beck J, Solomon A, Schmaman A: Gastroenteritis with necrotizing enterocolitis in premature babies. Brit Med J *2:* 616–619, 1972.
260. Sanders DY, Sinal SH, Morrison L: Chronic salmonellosis in infancy. Clin Pediat *13:* 640–643, 1974.
261. Marzetti G, Laurenti F, DeCaro M, Conca L, Orzalesi M: *Salmonella munchen* infections in newborns and small infants. An analysis of the clinical expression and manner of spread, as studies in two outbreaks. Clin Pediat *12:* 93–97, 1973.
262. Mayer JB: Appendicitis paratyphosa. Mitt a.d. Grenzgeb d. Med u. Chirg *43:* 550–556, 1934.
263. Hawkes SZ: Paratyphoid fever complicated by ruptured appendicitis. Ann Surg *110:* 466–472, 1939.
264. Seligmann E, Hertz JJ: Salmonella infections: report of 37 cases observed at Beth Israel Hospital, New York, in past 4 years. Ann Int Med *20:* 743–751, 1944
265. Rubenstein AD, Johnson BB: Salmonella appendicitis. Am J Med Sci *210:* 517–523, 1945.
266. Patel TB, Rao VN: Unusually high incidence of appendicitis cases at Dohad Town in Paneh Mahals District in Bombay State. Ind J Med Sci *12:* 517–520, 1958.
267. Meng GR: Acute mesenteric lymphadenitis due to *Salmonella enteritidis* mimicking appendicitis: Case report. Military Medicine *139:* 277, 1974.
268. Levine M: Cholecystitis due to *Salmonella oranienburg*: report of case with secondary wound infection. Minn Med *25:* 888, 1942.
269. Reisig G, Schaffner W: Postoperative detection of *Salmonella typhi*. Arch Surg *104:* 349–350, 1972.
270. Balows A: Unusual salmonella infections. J Kentucky State Med Assoc *56:* 770–773, 1958.

271. Harvey AM: *Salmonella suipestifer* infection in human beings: review of literature and report of twenty-one new cases. Arch Int Med *59:* 118–135, 1937.
272. Gadeholt H, Madsen ST: Clinical course, complications, and mortality in typhoid fever as compared with paratyphoid B. A survey of 2,647 cases. Acta Med Scand *174:* 753–760, 1963.
273. Marmion DE: The treatment of typhoid fever with chloramphenicol. Trans Roy Soc Trop Med Hyg *46:* 619–638, 1952.
274. Watson KC: Intravascular *Salmonella typhi* as a manifestation of the carrier state. Lancet *2:* 332–334, 1967.
275. Snyder MJ, Hornick AB, McCrumb FR Jr, Morse LJ, Woodward TE: Asymptomatic typhoidal bacteremia in volunteers. Antimicrob Agents Chemother *3:* 604–607, 1963.
276. Lehman JS Jr, Bassily S: Endotoxin tolerance in patients with chronic bacteremia and bacteriuria due to *Salmonella.* J Inf Dis *124:* 318–321, 1971.
277. Litwack KD, Hoke AW, Borchardt KA: Rose spots in typhoid fever. Arch Dermat *105:* 252–255, 1972.
278. Fraenkel E: Ueber Roseola typhosa. Z Hyg *34:* 481–494, 1900.
279. Gilman RH, Terminel M, Levine MM, Hernandez-Mendoza P, Hornick RB: Relative efficacy of blood, urine, rectal swab, bone-marrow, and rose-spot cultures for recovery of *Salmonella typhi* in typhoid fever. Lancet *1:* 1211–1213, 1975.
280. Top FH Sr: *Communicable and Infectious Diseases,* Sixth Edition, CV Mosby Co, St. Louis, 1968.
281. Dalrymple-Champneys W: *Brucella Infection and Undulant Fever in Man.* Oxford University Press, London, 1960.
282. Allen AC: *The Skin: A Clinicopathological Treatise.* Grune and Stratton Inc, New York, 1967.
283. Goscienski PJ, Haltalin KC: Rose spots associated with shigellosis. Am J Dis Child *119:* 152–154, 1970.
284. Gulati PD, Saxena SN, Gupta PS, Chuttani HK: Changing patterns of typhoid fever. Am J Med *45:* 544–548, 1968.
285. Wicks ACB, Holmes GS, Davidson L: Endemic typhoid fever; a diagnostic pitfall. Quart J Med *40:* 341–354, 1971.
286. Kim JP, Oh SK, Jarrett F: Management of ileal perforation due to typhoid fever. Ann Surg *181:* 88–91, 1975.
287. Mulligan TO: The treatment of typhoid perforations of the ileum. J Roy Coll Surg Edinburg *17:* 364–368, 1972.
288. Abdel-Meneim RI: Surgical management of perforated typhoid ulcer. Int Surg *52:* 405–410, 1967.
289. Dawson JH: Surgical management of typhoid perforation of the ileum. Amer Surg *36:* 620–622, 1970.
290. Rowland HAK: The complications of typhoid fever. J Trop Med Hyg *64:* 143–152, 1961.
291. Holmgren G: Severe intestinal hemorrhage in typhoid; a case report. Cent Afr J Med *19:* 267–269, 1973.
292. Poon MC, Sanders MG: Hepatic abscess caused by *Salmonella paratyphi* B. Canad Med Assoc J *107:* 529–531, 1972.
293. Faierman D, Ross FA, Seckler SG: Typhoid fever complicated by hepatitis, nephritis, and thrombocytopenia. JAMA *221:* 60–61, 1972.
294. Klatskin G: Hepatitis associated with systemic infections. *In* Schiff L (Ed): *Diseases of the Liver,* Third Edition, J. B. Lippincott Co, Philadelphia, 1969, pp. 602–644.
295. Ayhan A, Gokoz A, Karacadag S, Telatar H: The liver in typhoid fever. Am J Gastroenterol *59:* 141–146, 1973.
296. Ramachandran S, Godfrey JJ, Perera MVF: Typhoid hepatitis. JAMA *230:* 236–240, 1974.

297. Chuttani HK, Jain K, Misra RC: Small bowel in typhoid fever. Gut *12:* 709–712, 1971.
298. Shammaa MH, Ghazanafar SAS: D-xylose test in enteric fever, cirrhosis of the liver, and malabsorptive states. Brit Med J *2:* 836–838, 1960.
299. Crane RK: Intestinal absorption of sugars. Physiol Rev *40:* 789–825, 1960.
300. Russell IJ, Forgacs P, Geraci JE: Pancreatitis complicating typhoid fever; report of a case. JAMA *235:* 753–754, 1976.
301. DeMatteis A, Armani G: *Salmonella typhi* pneumonia without intestinal lesions. J Path Bact *94:* 464–467, 1967.
302. Thiruvengadam KV, Shetty MR, Mallick MA: Myocarditis in enteric fever. J Indian Med Assoc *48:* 115–119, 1967.
303. Rachmilewitz M, Braun K: Electrocardiographic changes in typhoid fever and their reversibility following niacin treatment. Am Heart J *36:* 284–294, 1948.
304. Mainzer F: Electrocardiographic study of typhoid myocarditis. Brit Heart J *9:* 145–153, 1947.
305. Diem LV, Arnold K: Typhoid fever with myocarditis. Am J Trop Med Hyg *23:* 218–221, 1974.
306. Eliakim M: Electrocardiographic signs of pericarditis in typhoid fever. Am J Med Sci *239:* 492–497, 1960.
307. Machiz S, Gordon J, Block N, Politano VA: *Salmonella typhosa* urinary tract infection and xanthogranulomatous pyelonephritis. J Fla Med Assoc *61:* 703–705, 1974.
308. Raybaud A, Martel-Reison C: Le rein typhique. Quelques aspects nephrologiques des fievres typhoides. Mars Med *102:* 601–606, 1965.
309. Amerio A, Campese VM, Coratelli P: Glomerulonephritis in typhoid fever (abstract). Fifth International Congress Nephrology *316:* 62, 1972.
310. Baker NM, Mills AE, Rachman I, Thomas JEP: Haemolytic-uraemic syndrome in typhoid fever. Brit Med J *2:* 84–87, 1974.
311. Riggall F, Salkind G, Spellacy W: Typhoid fever complicating pregnancy. Obstet Gyn *44:* 117–121, 1974.
312. Shaw AB: Haemoglobinuria in typhoid fever treated with chloramphenicol. Lancet *2:* 813–816, 1951.
313. Smith CEG: Haemoglobinuria in typhoid fever treated with chloramphenicol. Lancet *2:* 1020–1021, 1951.
314. McFadzean AJS, Choa GH: Haemolytic anemia in typhoid fever. Brit Med J *2:* 360–366, 1953.
315. Chatterji SC, Das PK: Chloramphenicol induced hemolytic anemia due to enzymatic deficiency of erythrocytes. J Ind Med Assoc *40:* 172–174, 1963.
316. Berry DH, Vietti TJ: Clinical manifestations of primaquine sensitive anemia. Am J Dis Child *110:* 166–171, 1965.
317. Robertson RP, Wahab MFA, Raasch FO: Evaluation of chloramphenicol and ampicillin in salmonella enteric fever. New Engl J Med *278:* 171–176, 1968.
318. Hersko C, Vardy PA: Haemolysis in typhoid fever in children with G-6-PD deficiency. Brit Med J *1:* 214–215, 1967.
319. Chan TK, Chesterman CN, McFadzean AJS, Todd D: The survival of glucose-6-phosphate dehydrogenase-deficient erythrocytes in patients with typhoid fever on chloramphenicol therapy. J Lab Clin Med *77:* 177–184, 1971.
320. McCaffrey RP, Halsted CH, Wahab MFA, Robertson RP: Chloramphenicol-induced hemolysis in Caucasian glucose-6-phosphate dehydrogenase deficiency. Ann Int Med *74:* 722–726, 1971.
321. Allen N, Nemanbhoy Y, Green D, Dunea G: Typhoid fever with consumption coagulopathy. JAMA *208:* 689–690, 1969.
322. Lehman JS Jr, Higashi GI, Bassily S, Farid Z: Rheumatoid factors in Salmonella and Schistosoma infections, Trans Roy Soc Trop Med *66:* 125–129,1972.

323. Leading Article: Psychiatric symptoms in typhoid fever, Brit Med J *2:* 436–437, 1973.
324. Osuntokun BO, Bademosi O, Ogunremi K, Wright SC: Neuropsychiatric manifestations of typhoid fever in 959 patients. Arch Neurol *27:* 7–13, 1972.
325. Ramachandran S, Wiekremesinghe HR, Perera MVF: Acute disseminated encephalomyelitis in typhoid fever. Brit Med J *1:* 494–495, 1975.
326. Vassa NT, Solanki SV, Yajnik VH: Myelitis due to enteric fever. Trop Geograph Med *25:* 245–248, 1973.
327. German GA, Arga OP: Psychiatric morbidity amongst a Uganda student population. Brit J Psych *115:* 1323–1329, 1969.
328. Chanmugan D, Waniganetti A: Guillain-Barre syndrome associated with typhoid fever. Brit Med J *1:* 95–96, 1969.
329. Mulligan TD: Typhoid fever in young children. Brit Med J *4:* 665–667, 1971.
330. Mani V, Brennand J, Mandal BK: Invasive illness with *Salmonella virchow* infection. Brit Med J *2:* 143–144, 1974.
331. Longcope WT: Paracolon infections, together with the report of a fatal case, with autopsy. Am J Med Sci *124:* 209–217, 1902.
332. Saphra I, Wassermann M: *Salmonella choleraesuis.* A clinical and epidemiological evaluation of 329 infections identified between 1940 and 1954 in the New York Salmonella Center. Am J Med Sci *228:* 525–533, 1954.
333. Allison MJ, Dalton HP, Escobar MR, Martin CJ: *Salmonella choleraesuis* infections in man: a report of 19 cases and a critical literature review. South Med J *62:* 593–596, 1969.
334. Goulder NE, Kingsland MF, Janeway CA: *Salmonella suipestifer* infection in Boston, a report of eleven cases, with autopsy findings in a case of bacterial endocarditis due to this organism and a study of the agglutination reactions in this infection. New Engl J Med *226:* 127–138, 1942.
335. Reichle FA, Tyson RR, Soloff LA, Lautsch EV, Rosemond GP: Salmonellosis and aneurysm of the distal abdominal aorta: case report with a review. Ann Surg *171:* 219–228, 1970.
336. Zak FG, Strauss L, Saphra I: Rupture of diseased large arteries in course of enterobacterial (Salmonella) infections. New Engl J Med *258:* 824–828, 1958.
337. Stengel A, Wolferth CC: Mycotic (bacterial) aneurysm of intravascular origin. Arch Int Med *31:* 527–554, 1923.
338. Rappaport BZ: Primary acute aortitis. Arch Path *2:* 653–658, 1926.
339. Parkhurst GF, Decker JP: Bacterial aortitis and mycotic aneurysm of aorta: report of 12 cases. Am J Path *31:* 821–835, 1955.
340. DeMuth WE Jr, McConaghie RJ: Salmonella infection in ruptured abdominal aortic aneurysm. Arch Surg *95:* 193–197, 1967.
341. Blum L, Keefer EBC: Clinical entity of cryptogenic mycotic aneurysm; report of 6 cases. JAMA *188:* 505–508, 1964.
342. Dehlinger KR: Salmonella osteomyelitis of spine associated with abdominal aortic aneurysm: report of a case. New Engl J Med *238:* 728–732, 1948.
343. Ten Eyck FW, Wellman WE: Salmonellosis associated with abdominal aortic aneurysm and edema of lower extremities: case report. Postgrad Med *26:* 334–339, 1959.
344. Bliss BP, Main RN, Scott JT: Ruptured abdominal aorta infected with *Salmonella brandenburg.* Brit Med J *4:* 751–752, 1968.
345. Silberman S, Greenblatt M: Primary mycotic aneurysm of the aorta; a complication of salmonellosis. Angiology *14:* 372–376, 1963.
346. Dixon RH, Lowicki EM: Salmonellosis associated with abdominal aortic aneurysm. South Med J *59:* 1403, 1408, 1966.
347. Lewis JF, Warshauer SE: Mycotic aneurysm of the abdominal aorta; a case due to *Salmonella choleraesuis var. Kunzendorf.* South Med J *62:* 597–598, 1969.
348. Bennett DE, Cherry JK: Bacterial infection of aortic aneurysms; a clinico-pathologic study. Am J Surg *113:* 321–326, 1967.

349. Meade RH III, Moran JM: Salmonella arteritis—preoperative diagnosis and cure of *Salmonella typhimurium* aortic aneurysm. New Engl J Med *281:* 310–312, 1969.
350. Mundth ED, Darling RC, Alvarado RH, Buckley MJ, Linton RR, Austen WG: Surgical management of mycotic aneurysms and the complications of infection in vascular reconstructive surgery. Am J Surg *117:* 460–470, 1969.
351. Kanwar YS, Malhotra V, Anderson BR, Pilz CG: Salmonellosis associated with abdominal aortic aneurysms. Arch Int Med *134:* 1095–1098, 1974.
352. Finseth F, Abbott WM: One-stage operative therapy for salmonella mycotic abdominal aortic aneurysm. Ann Surg *179:* 8–11, 1974.
353. Jarrett F, Darling RC, Mundth ED, Austen WG: Experience with infected aneurysms of the abdominal aorta. Arch Surg *110:* 1281–1286, 1975.
354. Abbott NE: Coarctation of the aorta of adult type. Am Heart J *3:* 574–618, 1928.
355. Buxton RW, Holdefer WF Jr: Primary mycotic aneurysms: review and report of a case. Amer Surg *29:* 863–867, 1963.
356. Barnett RN, Zimmerman SL: Coronary arteritis with total thrombosis due to *Salmonella cholesraesuis variety Kunzendorf.* Am Heart J *34:* 441–446, 1947.
357. Williams MJ: Perforating suppurative aortitis associated with idiopathic cystic medial necrosis. Am J Clin Path *22:* 160–165, 1952.
358. Weinstein L, Kaplan K: Salmonella aortitis in a patient with a Hufnagel valve. Circulation *31:* 755–758, 1965.
359. Yanoff M, Frank JH, Frost JW: Primary mycotic thoracic aortic aneurysm caused by *Salmonella choleraesuis.* Am J Med *38:* 145–150, 1965.
360. Crane AR: Primary multilocular mycotic aneurysm of aorta. Arch Path *24:* 634–641, 1937.
361. Simon SD, Silver CM: Salmonella osteomyelitis: report of three cases, one with fatal outcome and autopsy. J Int Surg *28:* 197–205, 1957.
362. MacCready RA, Reardon JP, Saphra I: Salmonellosis in Massachusetts: sixteen-year experience. New Engl J Med *256:* 1121–1128, 1957.
363. Cohen RA, Geraci JE, Dearing WH, Needham GM: Salmonellosis: observations on 94 patients. Mayo Clin Proc *39:* 401–409, 1964.
364. Weller C: Bacteremia due to *Salmonella choleraesuis variety Kunzendorf* (Paratyphoid C), complicated by ruptured aortic aneurysm. NY State J Med *52:* 1055–1056, 1952.
365. Schneider PJ, Nernoff J III, Gold JA: Acute salmonella endocarditis; report of a case and review. Arch Int Med *120:* 478–486, 1967.
366. Shilkin KB: *Salmonella typhimurium* pancarditis. Postgrad Med J *45:* 40–43, 1969.
367. Doraiswami S, Friedman SA, Kagan A, Gladstone JL: Salmonella endocarditis complicated by a myocardial abscess. Am J Card *26:* 102–105, 1970.
368. Geraci JE, Dearing WH: *Salmonella panama* endocarditis cured with kanamycin therapy. Proc Mayo Clinic *37:* 552–560, 1962.
369. Nushan HM, Sawyer CG, Rogers RO, Whitley NO: Bacterial endocarditis due to *Salmonella typhimurium.* Am J Card *7:* 608–612, 1961.
370. McNally EM, Kennedy RJ, Grace WR: *Salmonella infantis* infection of a preexistent ventricular aneurysm. Am Heart J *68:* 541–548, 1964.
371. Decker JP, Clancy CF: Salmonella endocarditis: report of three cases including one of mural endocarditis. Bull Ayer Clin Lab *4:* 1–5, 1959.
372. Connelly GP, Matthay RA, Sponzo RW, Smith FE: *Salmonella typhimurium* abscess formation in a calcified ventricular aneurysm. Chest *66:* 457–459, 1974.
373. Rubin RH, Moellering RC Jr: Clinical microbiologic, and therapeutic aspects of purulent pericarditis. Am J Med *59:* 68–78, 1975.
374. Weinstein L, Rubin RH: Infective endocarditis—1973. Prog Cardiovasc Dis *16:* 239–274, 1973.
375. Schatz JW, Wiener L, Gallagher HS, Eberly RJ: Salmonella pericarditis: An unusual complication of myocardial infection. Chest *64:* 267–269, 1973.

376. Langaker OM, Evans K: Myocardial abscess due to *Salmonella typhimurium*. Brit Heart J *35:* 871–873, 1973.
377. Tillotson JR, Lerner AM: Mycotic aneurysm and endocarditis; two uncommon complications of salmonella infection in the same patient. Am J Cardiol *18:* 267–274, 1966.
378. Danilowicz D, Posnock E, Chase R, Spencer FC: Salmonella septicemia after open heart surgery in an asymptomatic carrier. Am J Cardiol *34:* 864–867, 1974.
379. Svenbom M, Gastrin B, Rodriguez L: Transvenous cardiac pacemaker as a focus of salmonella infection in a patient with heart block. Acta Med Scand *196:* 281–284, 1974.
380. Joffe HS, Prosser GL, Chesler E, Schrire V: Salmonella endocarditis; successful treatment in childhood. Am J Dis Child *127:* 578–581, 1974.
381. Yamamoto N, Magidson O, Posner C, Mendez AM, Zubiate P, Kay JH: Probable salmonella endocarditis treated with prosthetic valve replacement: A case report. Surgery *76:* 678–681, 1974.
382. Paget J: On some of the sequels of typhoid fever. St. Bart's Hosp Rep *12:* 1–4, 1876.
383. Murphy JB: Bone and joint disease in relation to typhoid fever. Surg Gyn Obst *23:* 119–143, 1916.
384. Giacci L, Idriss H: Osteomyelitis due to salmonella infection, J Pediat *41:* 73–78, 1952.
385. White G, Meynell MJ: Paratyphoid-C: osteomyelitis of tibia. Lancet *1:* 362–363, 1956.
386. Hodges FJ, Holt JF: Editorial comment. *In* Hodges FJ et al. (Ed): *The 1951 Yearbook of Radiology,* Yearbook Publishers, Chicago, 1951, pp. 89.
387. Blanche DW: Osteomyelitis in infants. J Bone Joint Surg *34:* 71–84, 1952.
388. Kessel AWL: Acute osteomyelitis. Brit Med J *1:* 1352–1353, 1956.
389. Shaldlin B: Acute haematogenous osteomyelitis: a review of 300 cases treated during 1952–1959. South Afr Med J *34:* 520–524, 1969.
390. Waldvogel FA, Medoff G, Swartz MN: *Osteomyelitis: clinical features, therapeutic considerations and unusual aspects.* Charles C Thomas, Springfield, Ill., 1971, pp. 110.
391. Gajzago D, Gottche O: *Salmonella suipestifer* infections in childhood. Am J Dis Child *63:* 15–29, 1942.
392. David JR, Black RL: Salmonella arthritis. Medicine *39:* 385–403, 1960.
393. Hunt DD: Cervical spondylitis caused by *Salmonella oranienburg.* J Bone Joint Surg *47:* 1243–1246, 1965.
394. Walker GF: Typhoid spine in a Nigerian with sickle hemoglobin. J Bone Joint Surg (Brit) *45:* 683–686, 1963.
395. Mansoor IA: Typhoid osteomyelitis of the calcaneus due to direct inoculation; a case report. J Bone Joint Surg *49:* 732–734, 1967.
396. Schein AJ: Late infection of healed Lane-plated fracture of femur by *Salmonella typhimurium*: Lane plate as *locus minoris resistentiae.* J Mt Sinai Hosp *9:* 154–159, 1942.
397. Langenskiold A, Riska EB: Haematogenous salmonella infection around a metal hip endoprosthesis. Acta Orthop Scand *38:* 220–225, 1967.
398. Berglof FI: Arthritis and intestinal infection. Acta Rheum Scand *9:* 141–149, 1963.
399. Vartiainen H, Hurri L: Arthritis due to *Salmonella typhimurium.* Acta Medica Scand *175:* 771–776, 1964.
400. Warren CPW: Arthritis associated with salmonella infections. Ann Rheum Dis *29:* 483–487, 1970.
401. Edwards PR, Bruner DW, Moran AB: Further studies on the occurrence and distribution of salmonella types in the U.S. J Inf Dis *83:* 220–231, 1948.
402. Ghon J: Bericht uber den XIV: Internationalen Kongress fur Hygiene und Demographie. Berlin *4:* 21–23, 1907.
403. Beene ML, Hansen AE, Fulton N: Salmonella meningitis: Recovery from meningitis due to *Salmonella sp.* (*type Montevideo*) with consideraton of the problem of salmonella meningitis. Am J Dis Child *82:* 567–573, 1951.
404. Riley HD, Deardoff M: Salmonella meningitis. J Okla State Med Assoc *55:* 10–18, 1962.

405. Rabinowitz SC, MacLeod NR: Salmonella meningitis. A report of three cases and review of the literature. Am J Dis Child *123:* 259–262, 1972.
406. Guthrie KJ, Montgomery GL: Infections with *Bacterium enteritidis* in infancy with triad of enteritis, cholecystitis, and meningitis. J Path Bact *49:* 393–409, 1939.
407. Curbelo AJ, Martinez-Cruz JA: Historia de la *Salmonella habana*. Arch Med Inf *10:* 170–175, 1941.
408. High RH, Spaulding EH: Human infection with *Salmonella panama*. Am J Dis Child *72:* 181–188, 1946.
409. Weinstein L: Infections of the central nervous system. *In: The Practice of Infectious Disease*. Landsberger Medical Books, New York, 1958, p. 341.
410. Zia M, Haggerty RJ: Neonatal meningitis. New Engl J Med *259:* 314–320, 1958.
411. Collins FM, MacKaness GB, Blanden RV: Infection immunity as the basis of resistance to salmonella infections. J Exp Med *124:* 601–619, 1966.
412. Otila E: Studies on cerebrospinal fluid in premature infants. Acta Paediat Scand *35* (Suppl 8): 3–100, 1948.
413. Henderson LL: Salmonella meningitis: report of 3 cases and review of 144 cases from literature. Am J Dis Child *75:* 351–375, 1948.
414. Berman PH, Banker BQ: Neonatal meningitis: A clinical and pathological study of 29 cases. Pediatrics *38:* 6–24, 1966.
415. Barrett GS, MacDermot J: Breast abscess: a rare presentation of typhoid. Brit Med J *2:* 628–629, 1972.
416. Burry VF, Beezley M: Infant mastitis due to gram-negative organisms. Am J Dis Child *124:* 735–736, 1972.
417. Nelson JD: Suppurative mastitis in infants. Am J Dis Child *125:* 458–459, 1973.
418. Carswell W, Magrath IT: Skin ulceration caused by *Salmonella dublin*. Brit Med J *1:* 331–332, 1973.
419. Mitchell RG: Urinary-tract infections caused by salmonellae. Lancet *1:* 1082–1083, 1965.
420. Kostalas G, Thomas E: Orchitis and testicular abscess formation as complications of *Salmonella virchow* gastroenteritis. Medical J Aust *2:* 769–770, 1973.
421. Lerner PI, Golden PF, Jane JA: Salmonella-infected subdural hematoma. Pediatrics *49:* 127–128, 1972.
422. Vetrovec GW, Warner JF: Infected subdural hematoma: three case reports involving gram-negative organisms. Am J Med Sci *269:* 113–115, 1975.
423. Hirschman SZ, Murphy S: Peritonitis due to *Salmonella typhimurium* complicating nutritional cirrhosis. Mt Sinai J Med *38:* 470–473, 1971.
424. Kune GA, Coster D: Typhoid pancreatic abscess. Med J Aust *1:* 417–418, 1972.
425. Brelje MC, Garcia-Bunnel R: Salmonella infection in an ovarian dermoid cyst in pregnancy; report of a case. Obstet Gyn *24:* 279–280, 1964.
426. Sanders V, Misanik LF: Salmonella myocarditis; report of a case with ventricular rupture. Am Heart J *68:* 682–685, 1964.
427. Han T, Sokel JE, Neter E: Salmonellosis in disseminated malignant disease: a 7 year review (1959–1965). New Engl J Med *276:* 1045–1052, 1967.
428. Han T, Ezdinli EZ, Netter E: Chronic salmonella bacteriuria complicating lymphosarcoma. Am J Clin Path *54:* 837–838, 1970.
429. Wolfe MS, Armstrong D, Louria DB, Blevins A: Salmonellosis in patients with neoplastic disease; a review of 100 episodes at Memorial Cancer Center over a 13-year period. Arch Int Med *128:* 546–554, 1971.
430. Marr JJ, Haff RC: Superinfection of an amoebic abscess by *Salmonella enteritidis*. Arch Int Med *128:* 291–294, 1971.
431. Hahne OH: Lung abscess due to *Salmonella typhi*. Am Rev Resp Dis *89:* 566–571, 1964.
432. Sharr MM: Splenic abscess due to *Salmonella agona*. Brit Med J *1:* 546, 1972.

433. Curreri PW, Coller JA, MacVaughn H III: Subphrenic abscess secondary to salmonellosis. Arch Surg *95:* 189–192, 1967.
434. O'Neill JA Jr, Hall WH: Isolated adrenal abscess secondary to salmonellosis. Arch Surg *90:* 454–456, 1965.
435. Annamala A, Shreekumar S, Muthukumaran R: Empyema in enteric fever due to *Salmonella paratyphi B.* Dis Chest *55:* 72–74, 1969.
436. Abeloff MD, Densen P, Lenhard RE Jr: Salmonella empyema and Hodgkin's Disease. South Med J *68:* 636–639, 1975.
437. David DS, Brennan L, Grieco MH: Gas production with *Salmonella typhimurium* infection. Am J Med Sci *262:* 255–260, 1971.
438. Bille B, Mellbin T, Nordbring F: An extensive outbreak of gastroenteritis caused by *Salmonella newport.* Acta Med Scand *175:* 557–567, 1964.
439. Mellbin T, Nordbring F, Bille B: An extensive outbreak of gastroenteritis caused by *Salmonella newport.* III. Some clinical observations on 448 hospitalized cases and the results of cultures. Acta Med Scand *177:* 437–444, 1965.
440. Savage W: Problems of salmonella food poisoning. Brit Med J *2:* 317–321, 1956.
441. Gay FP: *Typhoid Fever.* MacMillan Company, New York, 1918, pp. 286.
442. Garbat AL: Typhoid carriers and typhoid immunity. *Omnis typhus ex typho.* Monograph 16 of the Rockefeller Institute for Medical Research, New York, 1922, pp. 1–110.
443. Ames WR, Robins M: Age and sex as factors in development of typhoid carrier state, and method for estimating carrier prevalence. Am J Public Health *33:* 221–230, 1943.
444. Thomson S: The number of bacilli harboured by enteric carriers. J Hyg *52:* 67–70, 1954.
445. Sharp JCM, Brown PP, Sangster G: Outbreak of paratyphoid in the Edinburgh area. Brit Med J *1:* 1282–1285, 1964.
446. Shaughnessy HJ, Freiwer F, Snyder A: Comparative efficiency of rectal swabs and fecal specimens in detecting typhoid and salmonella cases and carriers. Am J Public Health *38:* 670–675, 1948.
447. Feemster RF, Smith HM: Laboratory criteria of the cure of typhoid carrier. Am J Public Health *35:* 368–372, 1945.
448. Musher DM, Rubenstein AD: Permanent carriers of nontyphosa salmonellae. Arch Int Med *132:* 869–872, 1973.
449. Tynes BS, Utz JP: Factors influencing the cure of salmonella carriers. Ann Int Med *57:* 871–882, 1962.
450. Marselis JG Jr, Kaye D, Connolly CS, Hook EW: Quantitative bacteriology of the typhoid carrier state. Am J Trop Med *13:* 425–429, 1964.
451. Dinbar A, Altmann G, Tulcinsky DB: The treatment of chronic biliary salmonella carriers. Am J Med *47:* 236–242, 1969.
452. Waldram R, Vahrman J, Williams R: *Salmonella heidelberg* infection in *Caroli's Syndrome.* Gastroenterol 68: 151–153, 1973.
453. Melzer M, Altmann G, Rakowszcyk M, Yosipovitch ZH, Barsilia B: Salmonella infections of the kidney. J Urol *94:* 23, 27, 1965.
454. Hathout SE, El-Ghaffar YA, Awny AY, Hassan K: Relation between urinary schistosomiasis and chronic enteric urinary carrier state among Egyptians. Am J Trop Med *15:* 156–161, 1966.
455. Bassily S, Farid Z, Lehman JR Jr, Kent DC, Sanborn WR, Hathout SD: Treatment of chronic urinary salmonella carriers. Trans Roy Soc Trop Med Hyg *64:* 723–729, 1970.
456. Eisenberg GM, Palazzola AJ, Flippin HF: Clinical and microbiologic aspects of salmonellosis: study of ninety-five cases in adults and children. New Engl J Med *253:* 90–94, 1955.
457. Schneirson SS, Herschberger C, Honigsbery R: Salmonellosis at Mount Sinai Hospital: ten year survey (1953–1963). J Mt Sinai Hosp *31:* 1–9, 1964.

458. Hook EW: Salmonellosis: certain factors influencing interaction of salmonella and human host. Bull NY Acad Med *37:* 499–512, 1961.
459. Cherubin CE, Fodor T, Denmark LI, Master CS, Fuerst HT, Winter JW: Symptoms, septicemia and death in salmonellosis. Am J Epid *90:* 285–291, 1969.
460. Hook EW, Campbell CG, Weens HS, Cooper GR: Salmonella osteomyelitis in patients with sickle cell anemia. New Engl J Med *257:* 403–407, 1957.
461. Hendrickse RG, Collard P: Salmonella osteitis in Nigerian children. Lancet *1:* 80–82, 1960.
462. Ebrahim GJ, Grech P: Salmonella osteomyelitis in infants. J Bone Joint Surg (Brit) *48:* 350–353, 1966.
463. Diggs LW: Bone and joint lesions in sickle-cell disease. Clin Orth *52:* 119–143, 1967.
464. Weiss H, Katz S: Salmonella paravertebral abscess and cervical osteomyelitis in sickle-thalassemia disease. South Med J *63:* 339–341, 1970.
465. Van Oye E, Vassiliadis P: Osteomylite a Salmonella et hemoglobinopathie. *In* Van Oye E (Ed.): *The World Problem of Salmonellosis.* Monographiae Biologica, Vol XIII. The Hague, W Junk, 1964, pp. 232–242.
466. Specht EE: Hemoglobinopathic salmonella osteomyelitis; orthopedic aspects. Clin Orth *79:* 110–118, 1971.
467. Engh CA, Hughes JL, Abrams RC, Bowerman JW: Osteomyelitis in the patient with sickle-cell disease; diagnosis and management. J Bone Joint Surg *53:* 1–15, 1971.
468. Robbins JB, Pearson HA: Normal response of sickle cell anemia patients to immunization with salmonella vaccines. J Pediat *66:* 877–882, 1965.
469. Hook EW, Kaye D, Gill FA: Factors influencing host resistance to salmonella infection. The effects of hemolysis and erythrophagocytosis. Trans Amer Clin Climat Assoc *78:* 230–241, 1967.
470. Kaye D, Hook EW: The influence of hemolysis or blood loss on susceptibility to salmonella infection; additional observations. J Immun *91:* 65–75, 1963.
471. Kaye D, Hook EW: The influence of hemolysis on susceptibility to salmonella infection; additional observations. J Immun *91:* 518–527, 1963.
472. Kaye D, Hook EW: Influence of autoimmune hemolytic anemia on susceptibility to salmonella infection. Proc Soc Exp Biol Med *117:* 20–23, 1964.
473. Gill FA, Kaye D, Hook EW: The influence of erythrophagocytosis on the interaction of macrophages and salmonella *in vitro.* J Exper Med *124:* 173–183, 1966.
474. Kaye D, Gill FA, Hook EW: Factors influencing host resistance to salmonella infections: the effects of hemolysis and erythrophagocytosis. Am J Med Sci *254:* 205–215, 1967.
475. Giglioli G: *Paratyphoid C,* epidemic disease of British Guiana: clinical and pathological outline: *B. partyphosuim C,* a pyogenic organism: case reports. Proc Roy Soc Med *23:* 167–177, 1929.
476. Anderson TR, Zimmerman LE: Relapsing fever in Korea: clinico-pathologic study of 11 fatal cases with special attention to association with salmonella infections. Am J Path *31:* 1083–1109, 1955.
477. Ricketts WE: Intercurrent infections of Carrion's disease observed in Peru. Am J Trop Med Hyg *28:* 437–451, 1948.
478. Ricketts WE: Clinical manifestations of Carrion's disease. Arch Int Med *84:* 751–781, 1949.
479. Cuadra MC: Salmonellosis complication in human bartonellosis. Texas Rep Biol Med *14:* 97–113, 1956.
480. Sinkovics JG, Smith JP: Salmonellosis complicating neoplastic diseases. Cancer *24:* 631–636, 1969.
481. Gray LA: *Salmonella suipestifer* infection in myoma of uterus: report of case. Bull Johns Hopkins Hosp *59:* 231–236, 1936.
482. Graham FO, Coleman PN: Infection of secondary carcinoma by *Salmonella montevideo.* Brit Med J *1:* 1116, 1952.

483. Giel CP: Abscess formation in pheochromocytoma: report of case due to *Salmonella typhimurium*. New Engl J Med *251:* 980–982, 1954.
484. Patrizio RJ: Carcinoma of rectum as focus of *Salmonella bareilly* infection: report of case. J Intern Coll Surg *26:* 359, 1956.
485. Heineman HS, Jensen WN, Cooper WM, Braude AI: Hodgkin's disease and *Salmonella typhimurium* infection. JAMA *188:* 632–634, 1964.
486. Bowen ST, Gowen JW, Tauber OE: Cortisone and mortality in mouse typhoid. I. Effect of hormone dosage and times of injection. Proc Soc Exp Biol Med *94:* 476–479, 1957.
487. Hammond CW, Tompkins M, Miller CP: Occurrence of generalized infection of enteric origin in mice poisoned with nitrogen mustard. Proc Soc Exp Biol Med *82:* 137–140, 1953.
488. Shachmeister IL, Paulissen LJ, Fishman M: Sub-lethal total body x-irradiation and susceptibility of mice to *Salmonella enteritidis* and *Escherichia coli*. Proc Soc Exp Biol Med *83:* 205–209, 1953.
489. Farid Z, Bassily S, Kent DC, Sanborn WR, Hassan A, Abdel-Wahab MF, Lehman JS Jr: Chronic urinary salmonella carriers with intermittent bacteraemia. J Trop Med Hyg *73:* 153–156, 1970.
490. Bassily S, Farid Z, Lehman JS Jr, Ayad N, Sippel J: Treatment of chronic urinary salmonella carriers with trimethoprim-sulphamethoxazole. J Trop Med Hyg *75:* 227–229, 1972.
491. Tai Tze-Ying, Hsu Chao-Yueh, Chang Hsiao-Chih, Liu Yo Kun: Typhoid and paratyphoid fevers occurring in schistosomiasis. Chinese Med J *76:* 426–435, 1958.
492. Neves J, Lobo Martins NRDL: Long duration of septicaemic salmonellosis: 35 cases with 12 implicated species of salmonella. Trans Roy Soc Trop Med Hyg *61:* 541–552, 1967.
493. Neves J, Raso P, Marinho RP: Prolonged septicemic salmonellosis intercurrent with *Schistosomiasis mansoni* infection. J Trop Med Hyg *74:* 9–18, 1971.
494. Rocha H, Kirk JW, Heaney CD Jr: Prolonged salmonella bacteremia in patients with *Schistosoma mansoni* infection. Arch Int Med *128:* 254–257, 1971.
495. Farid Z, Higashi G, Bassily S, Young SW, Sparks HA: Chronic salmonellosis, urinary schistosomiasis, and massive proteinuria. Am J Trop Med Hyg *21:* 578–581, 1972.
496. Ottens H, Dickerson G: Bacterial invasion of schistosomes. Nature *223:* 506–507, 1969.
497. Leading Article: Biological control of schistosomiasis. Lancet *2:* 477–478, 1969.
498. Young SW, Higashi G, Kamel R: Schistosomes as the vehicles of salmonella infection. Trans Roy Soc Trop Med Hyg (abstract) *67:* 437, 1973.
499. Young SW, Higashi G, Kamel R, El Abdin AZ, Mikhail IA: Interactions of salmonellae and schistosomes in host-parasite relations. Trans Roy Soc Trop Med Hyg *67:* 797–802, 1973.
500. Neves J, Marinho RP, Martins NRLL, DeAraujo PK, Lucciola J: Prolonged septicaemic salmonellosis: treatment of intercurrent schistosomasis with niridazole. Trans Roy Soc Trop Med Hyg *63:* 79–84, 1969.
501. Lindeman RJ, Weinstein L, Levitan R, Patterson JF: Ulcerative colitis and intestinal salmonellosis. Am J Med Sci *254:* 855–861, 1967.
502. Banks B, Korelitz B, Zetzel L: The course of nonspecific ulcerative colitis: review of twenty years experience and late results. Gastroenterol *32:* 983–1012, 1957.
503. Dronfield MW, Fletcher J, Langman MJS: Coincident salmonella infections and ulcerative colitis: problems of recognition and management. Brit Med J *1:* 99–100, 1974.
504. Woodward TE, Smadel JE, Ley HL Jr, Green R, Mankakan DS: Preliminary report on the beneficial effect of chloromycetin in the treatment of typhoid fever. Ann Int Med *29:* 131–134, 1948.
505. Woodward TE, Smadel JE, Parker RT, Wisseman CL Jr: Treatment of typhoid fever with antibiotics. Ann NY Acad Sci *55:* 1043–1055, 1952.
506. Dawkins AT Jr, Hornick RB: Evaluation of antibiotics in a typhoid model. Antimicrob Agents Chemother *6:* 6–10, 1966.

507. Walker W: Cephaloride in typhoid. Brit Med J *2:* 1529–1530, 1964.
508. Holloway WJ, Scott EG: Clinical experience with cephaloridine. Antimicrob Agents Chemother *6:* 916–921, 1966.
509. Hermans PE, Martin JK Jr, Needham GM, Nichols DR: Laboratory and clinical evaluation of cephaloridine, a cephalosporin derivative. Antimicrob Agents Chemother *6:* 879–887, 1966.
510. Riley HD Jr, Ryan NJ: Failure of kanamycin in the treatment of typhoid fever. J Pediat *59:* 248–255, 1961.
511. Nelson JD, Haltalin KC: *In vitro* susceptibility of *E. coli,* shigellae, and salmonellae to kanamycin and therapeutic implications. Ann NY Acad Sci *132:* 1006–1014, 1966.
512. Sanford JP, Linh NN, Kutscher E, Arnold K, Gould K: Oxolinic acid in the treatment of typhoid fever due to chloramphenicol-resistant strains of *Salmonella typhi.* Antimicrob Agents Chemother *9:* 387–392, 1976.
513. Woodward TE, Smadel JE: Management of typhoid fever and its complications. Ann Int Med *60:* 144–157, 1964.
514. Scioli C, Giusti G, Balestrieri G: Comparison of ampicillin and chloramphenicol in treatment of paratyphoid fever. Brit Med J *1:* 148–150, 1964.
516. Patel KM: Ampicillin in typhoid fever, Brit Med J *1:* 907, 1964.
517. Manriquez L, Salcedo M, Borgono JM, Marzullo E, Kraljevic R, Paredes L, Valdivieso R: Clinical trials with ampicillin in typhoid fever and paratyphoid A. Brit Med J *2:* 152–153, 1965.
518. Sanders WL: Treatment of typhoid fever: a comparative trial of ampicillin and chloramphenicol. Brit Med J *2:* 1226–1227, 1965.
519. Kaye D, Rocha H, Eyckmans L, Prata A, Hook EW: Comparison of parenteral ampicillin and parenteral chloramphenicol in the treatment of typhoid fever. Ann NY Acad Sci *145:* 423–428, 1967.
520. Wahab MFA, Robertson RP, Raasch FO: Paratyphoid A fever. Ann Int Med *70:* 913–917, 1969.
521. Mikhail IA, Kent DC, Sorensen K, Sanborn WR, Smith J: Concentrations of ampicillin and chloramphenicol in the serum of patients with acute *Salmonella* enteric fever. Antimicrob Agents Chemother *2:* 336–339, 1972.
522. Calderon E: Amoxicillin in the treatment of typhoid fever due to chloramphenicol-resistant *Salmonella typhi.* J Inf Dis *129* (Suppl): S219–S221, 1974.
523. Munnich D, Bekesi S, Lakatos M, Bardovics E: Treatment of typhoid carriers with amoxycillin and in combination with probenecid. Chemotherapy *20:* 29–38, 1974.
524. Pillay N, Adams EB, North-Coombes D: Comparative trial of amoxycillin and chloramphenicol in treatment of typhoid fever in adults. Lancet *2:* 333–334, 1975.
525. Scragg JN, Rubidge CJ: Amoxycillin in treatment of typhoid fever in children. Am J Trop Med Hyg *24:* 860–865, 1975.
526. Gilman RH, Terminel M, Levine MM, Hernandez-Mendosa, Calderone E, Vasquez V, Martinez E, Snyder MJ, Hornick RB: Comparison of trimethoprim-sulfamethoxazole and ampicillin in therapy of chloramphenicol-resistant and chloramphenicol-sensitive typhoid fever. J Inf Dis *132:* 630–636, 1975.
527. Akinkugbe VO, Lewis EA, Montefiore D, Okubadejo OA: Trimethoprim and sulphamethoxazole in typhoid. Brit Med J *3:* 721–722, 1968.
528. Farid Z, Hassan A, Wahab MFA, Sanborn WR, Kent DC, Yassa A, Hathout SE: Trimethoprim-sulphamethoxazole in enteric fevers. Brit Med J *3:* 323–324, 1970.
529. Kamat SA: Evaluation of therapeutic efficacy of trimethoprim-sulphamethoxazole and chloramphenicol in enteric fever. Brit Med J *3:* 320–322, 1970.
530. Leading Article: Trimethoprim-sulphamethoxazole in typhoid. Brit Med J *3:* 297–298, 1970.
531. Geddes AM, Fothergill R, Goodall JAD, Dorken PR: Evaluation of trimethoprimsul-

phamethoxazole compound in treatment of salmonella infection. Brit Med J *3:* 451–454, 1971.

532. Saudesai HV, Melinkere RD, Diwate AB: Trimethoprim-sulphamethoxazole in typhoid fever. Trans Roy Soc Trop Med Hyg *65:* 189–194, 1971.
533. Scragg JN, Rubidge CJ: Trimethoprim and sulphamethoxazole in typhoid fever in children. Brit Med J *3:* 738–741, 1971.
534. Franzen C, Lidin-Janson G, Nygren B: Trimethoprim-sulphamethoxazole in enteric infections. Scand J Inf Dis *4:* 231–240, 1972.
535. Marks MI, Kazemi M, Mackay E: *In vitro* sensitivity of *Salmonella* to ten antimicrobial agents including sulfamethoxazole and trimethoprim, alone and in combination. Antimicrob Agents Chemother *4:* 555–559, 1973.
536. Kazemi M, Gumpert TG, Marks MI: A controlled trial comparing sulfamethoxazole-trimethoprim, ampicillin, and no therapy in the treatment of salmonella gastroenteritis in children. J Pediat *83:* 646–650, 1973.
537. Snyder MJ, Perroni J, Gonzalez O, Palomino C, Gonzalez C, Music S, DuPont HL, Hornick RB, Woodward TE: Trimethoprim-sulfamethoxazole in the treatment of typhoid and paratyphoid fevers. J Inf Dis *128* (Suppl): S734–S737, 1973.
538. Lurie I, Felner S, Burke M: The value of trimethoprim-sulfamethoxazole in the treatment of *Salmonella* infections. Israel J Med Sci *10:* 1420–1424, 1974.
539. Marks MI: Pharmacokinetics and efficacy of trimethoprim-sulfamethoxazole in the treatment of gastroenteritis in children. Canad Med Assoc J *112:* (13 Special #): S33–S34, 1975.
540. Geddes AM: Trimethoprim-sulfamethoxazole in the treatment of gastrointestinal infections, including enteric fever and typhoid carriers. Canad Med Assoc J *112* (13 Special #): S35–S36, 1975.
541. DuPont HL, Hornick RB, Weiss CF, Snyder MJ, Woodward TE: Evaluation of chloramphenicol acid succinate therapy of induced typhoid fever and Rocky Mountain spotted fever. New Engl J Med *282:* 53–57, 1970.
542. Coles H, Stewart GT: Current therapeutics—paromomycin. Practitioner *186:* 379–387, 1961.
543. Joint Project by Members of the Association for the Study of Infectious Diseases: Effect of neomycin in non-invasive salmonella infections of the gastrointestinal tract. Lancet *2:* 1159–1161, 1970.
544. Pettersson T, Klemola E, Wager O: Treatment of acute cases of salmonella infection and salmonella carriers with ampicillin and neomycin. Acta Med Scand *175:* 185–190, 1964.
545. Aserkoff B, Bennett JV: Effect of antibiotic therapy in acute salmonellosis on the fecal excretion of salmonellae. New Engl J Med *281:* 636–640, 1969.
546. Dixon JMS: Effect of antibiotic treatment on duration of excretion of *Salmonella typhimurium* by children. Brit Med J *2:* 1343–1345, 1965.
547. Rosenthal SL: Exacerbation of salmonella enteritis due to ampicillin. New Engl J Med *280:* 147–148, 1969.
548. Smith ER, Badley BWD: Treatment of salmonella enteritis and its effect on the carrier state. Canad Med Assoc J *104:* 1004–1006, 1971.
549. Szanton V: Epidemic salmonellosis: A 30 month study of 80 cases of *Salmonella oranienburg* infection. Pediat *20:* 794–808, 1957.
550. Mandell GL, Hook EW: Persistence of ampicillin-sensitive *Salmonella thompson* due to fecal penicillinase. Arch Int Med *127:* 137–138, 1971.
551. Bessudo D, Heredia Duarte A, Bucio R: Rifampicin in eradication of salmonella from the intestinal tract. Chemotherapy *17:* 71–78, 1972.
552. Nalin DR, Cash RA, Islam R, Molla M, Phillips RA: Oral maintenance therapy for cholera in adults. Lancet *2:* 370–373, 1968.

553. Nalin DR, Cash RA, Rahman M, Junus M: Effect of glycine and glucose on sodium and water absorption in patients with cholera. Gut *11:* 768–772, 1970.
554. WHO: Principles and practice of cholera control. *Public Health Papers* No. 40, WHO, Geneva, 1970.
555. Cash RA, Nalin DR, Rochat R, Reller LB, Haque ZA, Rahman ADMM: A clinical trial of oral therapy in a rural cholera treatment center. Am J Trop Med Hyg *19:* 653–656, 1970.
556. Cash RA, Nalin DR, Forrest JN, Abrutyn E: Rapid correction of acidosis and dehydration of cholera with oral electrolyte and glucose solution. Lancet *2:* 549–550, 1970.
557. Leading Article: Oral glucose-electrolyte therapy for acute diarrhea. Lancet *1:* 79–80, 1975.
558. Rohde JE, Northrup RS: Taking science where the diarrhoea is. *In,* Acute Diarrhoea in Children, Ciba Foundation Symposium 42, American Elsevier, New York, 1976, pp. 339–366.
559. Harries JT: The problem of bacterial diarrhoea. *In,* Acute Diarrhoea in Children, Ciba Foundation Symposium 42, American Elsevier, New York, 1976, pp. 3–25.
560. Field M: Regulation of active ion transport in the small intestine. *In,* Acute Diarrhoea in Children, Ciba Foundation Symposium 42, American Elsevier, New York, 1976, pp. 109–127.
561. Wisseman CL, Paterson PY, Smadel J, Diercks F, Ley HL Jr: Studies on cortisone and antibiotics for prompt therapeutic control of typhoid fever and scrub typhus. J Clin Invest *33:* 264–275, 1954.
562. Holt R: The bacterial degradation of chloramphenicol. Lancet *1:* 1259–1260, 1967.
563. Robertson RP, Wahab MFA: Influence of chloramphenicol and ampicillin on antibody response in typhoid-paratyphoid fever. Ann Int Med *72:* 219–221, 1970.
564. Stamps TJ, Wicks ACB: Trimethoprim-sulfamethoxazole (Bactrim) in the treatment of typhoid fever. S African Med J *46:* 652–655, 1972.
565. Jaques PH, Van der Heyde H: Combination of trimethoprim and sulfamethoxazole in typhoid fever. S Afr Med J *46:* 281–284, 1972.
566. Olurin EO, Ajayi OD, Bohrer SP: Typhoid perforations. J Roy Coll Surg Edinburgh *17:* 353–363, 1972.
567. Angorn IB, Pillay SP, Hegarty M, Baker LW: Typhoid perforation of the ileum; a therapeutic dilemma. South Afr Med J *49:* 781–784, 1975.
568. Welch TP, Martin NC: Surgical treatment of typhoid perforation. Lancet *1:* 1078–1080, 1975.
569. Collins WJ, Ball RE, Dorsey TJ: Typhoid ileitis with hemorrhage; a case report with new therapy. Am J Dig Dis *20:* 94–96, 1975.
570. Birnholz JC: Primary salmonella mycotic aortic aneurysm. Report of a case diagnosed by radionuclide angiography. Vasc Surg *7:* 45–48, 1973.
571. Vogelsang TM: *Typhoid and Paratyphoid B Carriers and their Treatment: Experiences from Western Norway.* Grieg, Bergen, 368 pp., 1960.
572. Main RG: Treatment of chronic alimentary enteric carriers. Brit Med J *1:* 328–333, 1961.
573. Vogelsang TM: The campaign against typhoid and paratyphoid B in western Norway. Results of cholecystectomy. J Hyg *62:* 443–449, 1964.
574. Christie AB: Treatment of typhoid carriers with ampicillin. Brit Med J *1:* 1609–1611, 1964.
575. Whitby JMF: Ampicillin in treatment of *Salmonella typhi* carriers. Lancet *2:* 71–72, 1964.
576. Bullock WE: Ampicillin therapy of salmonella carriers: a summary of laboratory and clinical observations. Am J Med Sci *246:* 42–47, 1963.
577. Perkins JC, Devetsk RL, Dowling HF: Ampicillin in the treatment of salmonella carriers. Arch Int Med *118:* 528–533, 1966.
578. Russell EM, Sutherland A, Walker W: Ampicillin for persistent typhoid excreters, including a clinical trial in convalescence. Brit Med J *2:* 555–557, 1966.

579. Simon HJ, Miller RC: Ampicillin in the treatment of chronic typhoid carriers. New Engl J Med *274:* 807–815, 1966.

580. Kaye D, Merselis JG Jr, Connolly CS, Hook EW: Treatment of chronic enteric carriers of *Salmonella typhosa* with ampicillin. Ann NY Acad Sci *145:* 429–435, 1967.

581. Phillips WE: Treatment of chronic typhoid carriers with ampicillin. JAMA *217:* 913–915, 1971.

582. Johnson WD Jr, Hook EW, Lindsey E, Kaye D: Treatment of chronic typhoid carriers with ampicillin. Antimicrob Agents Chemother *3:* 439–440, 1973.

583. Scioli C, Fiorentino F, Sasso G: Treatment of *Salmonella typhi* carriers with intravenous ampicillin. J Inf Dis *125:* 170–173, 1972.

584. Brodie J, MacQueen IA, Livingstone D: Effect of trimethoprim-sulphamethoxazole on typhoid and salmonella carriers. Brit Med J *3:* 318–319, 1970.

585. Chan ACH, Forrest CR, Robertson MJ: A fourteen-day treatment of typhoid carriers in Hong Kong with trimethoprim-sulphamethoxazole. Med. J Aust *1:* 386–388, 1973.

586. Clementi KJ: Trimethoprim-sulfamethoxazole in the treatment of carriers of *Salmonella.* J Inf Dis *128* (Suppl): S738–S742, 1973.

587. Pichler H, Knothe H, Spitzy KH, Vielkind G: Treatment of chronic carriers of *Salmonella typhi* and *Salmonella paratyphi B* with trimethoprim-sulfamethoxazole. J Inf Dis *128* (Suppl): S743–S744, 1973.

Index